Ayurveda and Yoga –
Prevention and Self-Healing through Awareness

KLAUS-RUPPRECHT WASMUHT

Ayurveda and Yoga

Prevention and Self-Healing through Awareness

A small Guide for a fulfilling and happy Life

Translated from the German by Janette Marson

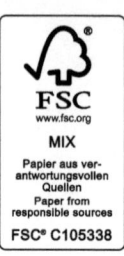

Bibliographical Information of the Deutsche Nationalbibliothek
This publication is listed in the Deutsche Nationalbibliographie of the
Deutsche Nationalbibliothek; detailed bibliographical information
can be accessed under http: //dnb.d-nb.de

© 2019 Klaus-Rupprecht Wasmuht
Translation © 2019 Janette Marson

Printing, production and layout:
Books on Demand GmbH. Norderstedt
ISBN: 978-3-7481-9488-0

Inhalt

Preliminary remarks   7

Prologue   11

1. Mesocosm   15
   Immensity of the universe   18
   Basic concepts: Vedanta and Sāṃkhya philosophy related to
   Ayurveda and Yoga   23
   Physical constitution and mental constitution   31

2. Modern medicine without soul?   37
   Evidence Based Medicine (EBM) of Ayurveda and Medicine
   Based Evidence (MBE) of Modern Medicine   40
   Psychosomatic medicine   43
   Placebo and Nocebo   44
   Socio-Psycho-Neuro-Endocrino-Immunology   47
   Interpersonal neurobiology - the social synapse   50

3. Consciousness - know yourself   52
   Moral crisis   52
   Spiritual development   53
   Mental functions in Ayurveda   56

4. Prevention and self-healing – Cornerstones of Ayurveda   60
   Health is contentment, illness is discontent   61
   Excursus regarding happiness, health, longevity: 62
   Swasthya – Rest in Self   69
   Recognizing causes of illness   72
   Assessment of some major diseases and ailments of the mind from the
   ayurvedic point of view   84

5. Ayurveda and Yoga- the magical connection of human life
with the immediate environment and the universe   98
    The first two limbs of the eight paths of Yoga (Patañjali –
    Ashtanga Yoga)   100

Epilogue   118

References   120

Vita   130

Preliminary remarks

This book is not intended to make diagnoses or to recommend prescriptions. The information contained herein is in no way to be considered as a substitute for consultation with a properly licensed healthcare professional.

This book is also not designed as a kind of manual and also does not claim to offer a systematic presentation.

In numerous ayurvedic and yoga handbooks translated into German, individual components of ayurvedic medicine and yoga have been described in great detail in the Western Hemisphere over the last few decades and detailed instructions, measures and rules of conduct for a healthy lifestyle are given.

These very readable sources report how body forces can be developed and promoted through, for example, physical exercises (asanas), breathing exercises, nutrition appropriate to the constitution, and much more. Interested readers may inform themselves by studying these works (see some sources) [1]

To merely supplement these would only serve to "embellish" without actually adding any real enrichment; that is not my intention.

Rather, this book is intended as a small guide, that may accompany the reader in his walk on the path of ayurvedic wisdom in conjunction with yoga. In this way, the reader may be encouraged to think and move forward consciously step by step.

With regard to yoga it should be noted at this stage that attention is paid first and foremost to the ethical principles of the first two elements of classical Ashtanga Yoga (Patanjeli Sutras), which is less well known in Western culture.
  To facilitate the understanding of ayurvedic and yogic wisdom, numerous comparisons are made which correspond to Western attitudes.

For me as the author of this book, it is more important to sketch the interlocking essentials than to present a detailed presentation.

Stage 1
The first guidance in the prologue is the need to eliminate ignorance. The key to this is offered by the symbolic content of the cosmic dance of god Shiva.

Stage 2
The following section "Mesocosm" intends to suggest the immensity of the Universe, and to discern man, insignificant as he may seem against this background as a highly evolved living spiritual being in an extremely complex relationship of interactions, both with his Inner world as well as with the Outer world.

Stage 3
Here is a reference to the oldest philosophical directions of Indian origin, in which already fundamental principles of ayurvedic healing and Yoga, such as consciousness, spirit, soul, natural elements and other factors of existence are expressed.

Stage 4
From the beginning, according to the ayurvedic teachings, the world consists of five elements (Pancha Boothas): space (Akash), air (Vayu), fire (Agni), water (Apas / Jal) and earth (Prithvi).

They determine everything: the essence of stones, plants, animals and humans. Man is between microcosm and macrocosm as mesocosm of the world. All elements are also found in his body, for example in his five senses: in listening (space), in seeing (fire), in smelling (earth), in feeling (air) and in tasting (water).

The physical constitution (Dosha) Vata, Pitta, Kapha sheds light on the basic bio-physical structure, which is differently distributed in each person. The knowledge of one's own constitution also makes it possible to recognize the difference of one's fellow man. With this understanding may also be brought more tolerance for the differences in fellow human beings.

Stage 5
In addition to the physical constitution, the spiritual constitution – Tri-Gunas (Sattva, Rajas, Tamas) – is of elementary importance in Ayurveda, both for the thinking, acting and well-being as well as for the conscious life development of humans.

The properties of Tri-Gunas, such as sattva (light, clarity), rajas (activity, movement), and tamas (inertia, darkness) were first systematized in Samkhya philosophy and later considered in Vedanta.

They are also interpreted on the cosmic level as subtle matter. They form the qualitative properties of primal matter (prakriti).

In contrast to the doshas, which are already determined at the conception, a certain development is possible with the Gunas. This can take place in an expansion of consciousness and spiritual development, expressed in thought and action.

Therefore, the three gunas are also given special attention in yoga.

The yoga practitioner is encouraged to align his life from inertia to movement, from activity to clarity, and finally to transcend sattva.

The Bhagavadgita, interpreted by the Hindus as the quintessence of the Vedas, describes in detail in the fourteenth, seventeenth, and eighteenth chapters the elemental meaning of the gunas for man.

Stage 6
A consideration of body, mind and soul is introduced here as we look towards modern medicine and the issue "medicine without soul". This complex topic has been heavily disputed since ancient times and culminated in the Cartesian ontology in the separation of body and soul.

I do not join in this controversy, but comment briefly on areas of placebo / nocebo, psychosomatics and more recent research areas of socio-psycho-neuro-endocrino immunology and interpersonal neurobiology.

In particular, the interactions between negative and positive mental factors on the immune system in connection with the particular importance in Ayurveda and Yoga should be looked at a bit closer in the later section "Health and Disease" and in the final chapter.

Stage 7
Having arrived at this point, a deliberate engagement with the SELF appears to be appropriate, as opposed to the "I", to pay attention to one of the key issues of Ayurveda and Yoga.

Depending on the depth of his awareness, man lives in coarse form (tamas), in lively form (rajas), or in self-confident form (sattva).

Resting in the self ("swasthya") not only means being free of illness, but being in sensual clarity, having mental and spiritual health and living spiritual fulfillment.

In short: sheltered in basic trust.

Stage 8
The path continues, now leading to prevention and self-healing.

Health care of Ayurveda deals predominantly with prevention of diseases. This is a fundamental difference to classical medicine!

The treatment of illnesses, also in terms of self-healing, will, of course, be given attention if, despite prevention, a disease is emerging.

Following on from the above-described effects of negative psychological factors on the immune system, some of the main illnesses and ailments of the mind with a focus on depressive disorders are evaluated here from an ayurvedic perspective. The various treatment methods presented here illustrate the complex holistic approach of ayurvedic medicine, which, at the same time, integrates physique, psyche and spirituality into one another.

Stage 9
After all this the magical connection of yoga and ayurveda is addressed again. Of particular importance here are effects of positive psychic factors on the immune system and the influence of the realization of ethical behavior on consciousness.

Yoga in the deeper sense means the expansion of one's consciousness and spiritual development and thus a perfection of human existence.

Epilogue
A review concludes the journey. May the reader contemplate, reflect, shaping an inner picture of the future in a vision that will fill him with confidence and lead him safely on his further path of life.

Prologue

The modern science of the Western world has found various means to enable a standard of living beyond the subsistence level. However, it has done little to facilitate inner self-realization and true emotional satisfaction. Greater material well-being is accompanied by a regrettable increase in mental illness, drug addiction, suicide, crime, corruption and violence.

In the Eastern world, on the other hand, human beings have developed emotional and spiritual techniques that lead to the realization of the connection with the metaphysical. The appropriate way of life has made it possible to free oneself from existential doubts and suffering internally. However, most people have so far failed to solve the urgent issues of everyday life and to improve their living conditions.[2]

Realization:
Material prosperity alone does not mean a happy life yet, and spiritual freedom in material distress does not provide sufficient livelihood.

Question:
In the social environment, how can one be connected to the other in order to enable a full and happy life in community?

The title page shows Shiva as Nataraja ("King of Dance") in the cosmic dance, dancing on Apasmara, the "Demon of Ignorance".
　　In dance, Shiva destroys ignorance

The essential meaning of Shiva's dance is threefold: First: it is the image of his rhythmic play as the source of all motion in the cosmos represented by the bow:
　　Second: the purpose of his dance is to remove the innumerable souls of men from the trap of illusion.
　　Third: the place of the dance, Chidambaram, is the center of the universe, in the heart.[3]

What does Shiva tell us as a symbol of the source of all movement in the cosmos – liberation from the trap of illusion – the heart as the center of the universe?

Liberation from the illusion is today desirable through self-realization.

Is not this desire already an expression of an illusion? Sri Ramana Maharshi [4] answers this question as follows: "The desire to realize the Self is at the same time an expression of a deficiency phenomenon. The very nature of this sense of life hides itself as a secret, the meaning of which only reveals itself to a few people."

This leads to the question: what is the actual character of this self-awareness of life, which hides itself as a secret and reveals itself to only a few people?
 What would life be like if humanity managed to solve this mystery?

Would the crew in "Spaceship Earth" be able to shape their coexistence in a cooperative team spirit, rather than in a competition-dictated "survival of the fittest"? In other words "keeping healthy" instead of "getting sick"!

Ayurveda and yoga – prevention and self-healing through awareness – are means to reveal and promote awareness of the true character of "this feeling for life", called "Swasthya" in Hinduism,

Swasthya, or rest in the self, is naturally devoid of pathological aspects. Only by misjudging the circumstances and subsequent misconduct problems appear that have a negative impact.

The cause of this sequence is a lack of knowledge, lack of awareness about the interactions of complex life processes and thus misguided lifestyle.

This ignorance or misjudgment in coexistence of people has led from the earliest beginnings to the present to social conflicts and armed conflicts in the political and religious environment, as well as in economic dealings and in many other areas of life.

The world has become a big village in the last decades, in a few hours every point of the earth can be reached. Have we become world citizens for that reason alone?
 Or do we see the events too much out of our own glasses, if not rose-tinted glasses, conditioned from early youth, shaped by the social environment, stubbornly blocked in dogmas and automatisms?

In this book, the ayurvedic approach is explained in connection with yoga, which is primarily preventive and health-promoting, taking into account the patient's own physical, mental and spiritual activity, focusing on awareness of self-ordering and self-healing interactions.

The desired shift from a purely curative to a preventive-curative medicine, and finally a medicine that primarily pursues the goal of prevention through health promotion, requires an understanding of complex holistic interactions, an understanding of individual dynamics, and an understanding of how a person's life has developed.

1. Mesocosm

Human being – Cosmic dust and what else? "

There are areas of life that we do not know about. However, when we apply to them the principle of analogy (in philosophy, a form of agreement on certain characteristics), we extend our understanding beyond these realms. The principle of analogy reveals itself as a universal law on various levels of the material, intellectual and spiritual universe.[5]

Already the spread of the galaxies seems gigantic to humans, an order of magnitude that can hardly be grasped, whereas atomic distances seem very tiny to humans.

Ultimately, this similarity of the different levels of existence is due to the mental state of consciousness.[6]

Mesocosm in philosophy is the subject area of objects clearly intelligible to human beings. This is understood as an intermediate area between microcosm and macrocosm.

The mesocosm is important in that it defines the range of perception from which humans can describe the macrocosm and the microcosm.[7]

Consciousness can be compared to the tip of an iceberg and the unconscious to the hidden much larger part of the iceberg.

The situation is similar with the sensory perception of man. Even a rough assessment of the human senses reveals the limitations to what we can see and hear.

Sound spectrum:

People can only hear vibrations with a frequency of 20 Hertz up to 16000 Hz (maximum 20000 Hz). Elephants, cattle and insects, on the other hand, hear very deep sounds whose sound waves propagate over long distances below 16 Hz. Pigeons can even hear sounds in the 0.1 Hertz range.

In the high frequency range, hedgehogs, dogs, dolphins and bats are superior to humans. Bats can hear sounds up to 200,000 hertz.

Apart from the sound phenomenon as a physical phenomenon, sound is of particular importance in numerous creation myths.

For Joachim-Ernst Berendt, the longtime jazz editor of Südwestfunk Baden Baden sound is the continuous principle of creation.(8)

He saw a harmonic principle not only in the music of all cultures, but also in nature (fauna and flora) and in space, in the orbits and vibrations of the planets.
  Oxygen particles vibrate in C major, the blades of a mountain meadow "sing", photosynthesis creates triads.

Berendt thought that Copernicus must be taken literally. God himself created the world out of sound, so reject all music to God or to the Gods.

The Bible emphasizes in several places the meaning of sound and light. "In the beginning was the Word, and the Word was with God, and the Word was God. [9] The same was in the beginning with God. All things are made by the same, and without it is nothing made that was made. [10]
  In him was life, and life was the light of men. (11) And the light shines in the darkness, and the darkness has not understood. [12]

According to Indian philosophy, the world is sound (Nada Brahma). The sound of Nada stands for the sacred syllable OM.[13] Om is the most sublime symbol of the Hindu Metaphysics.

As a transcendental primordial sound, OM refers to vibrations that created the entire universe. Om stands as sound for the beginning, without matter.

Building on this, the perceptible, the material universe emerged. So much is mentioned here to OM. Particular importance is given to the effect of OM-chanting in yoga practice for more awareness of body and mind, to recognize the Self and return to the essence of nature.[14]

According to Professor Klaus Fessmann, pianist, composer and sound artist, "Sound and music are vital. Sound and music not only reverse misery, but at the same time prevent fear." [15]

"When I was sitting in a circle with a group of ADHD children in the clinic of Esslingen with sound stones in a circle on the floor and we were playing, they suddenly knew what they had to do with their hands and their urge to move: they entered into the movement of the music of the stones, which was like them, like their senses and feelings, their being and their way of thinking.

They did not need any Ritalin, no therapies, prescriptions, or anything like that, just meaningful and fulfilling movements and accompanying notes in their Musica Humana."

Electromagnetic spectrum:

In the electromagnetic spectrum, the light spectrum with wavelengths between approximately 380 and 780 nm is the part visible to the human eye.

At the beginning of the spectrum are the short-wave and thus high-energy gamma rays whose wavelength reaches atomic magnitudes. At the end are the longitudinal waves whose wavelengths are many kilometers.

Light, like fire, is one of the most important phenomena of all human cultures. "Light casts no shadow."[16] The existence of the shadow is dependent on the light, but the light is not dependent on the shadow and can never be reached by the shadow.

Although only a limited portion of the electromagnetic spectrum is visible to the human physical eye, the "spiritual" eye has produced a much wider notion of light.

Thus mankind has made astonishing discoveries since fire was brought to mankind by Prometheus, who is considered the originator of human civilization.

In particular, the discovery of power generation in modern times enabled electric propulsion and power supply over long distances.

Classical electrodynamics has been extended by quantum electrodynamics (quantum field theory description of electromagnetism).

Nuclear energy also highlights the downsides of human activity: the A-bomb dropping on Hiroshima and Nagasaki, as well as the Chernobyl and Fukushima disasters - to name only the most monstrous derailments - have caused and still cause unspeakable suffering.

The following points of view, both scientific and spiritual, which are in line with the main message, seem more luminous. According to Frido Mann and Christine Mann, the authors of the book "Let Light Be: The Unity of Mind and Matter in Quantum Physics", [17] the change in natural sciences through quantum theory enables a holistic view of the world and of man in which contrast of idealism and materialism is overcome.

According to the spiritual teacher Chinmoy Kumar Ghose (known as Sri Chinmoy), the light adopts humanity with all its imperfections and seeks to enlighten human ignorance so that human life can become divine life.[18]

For more on the healing effects of light, see the final chapter: Ayurveda and Yoga.

Immensity of the universe

I consider the following to be particularly important in explaining to the interested reader how progressive the way of thinking of the ancient sages of India was several millennia ago, not only in the field of cosmology, but also in other fields of knowledge, such as in the field of medicine.

The allegedly modern medical science, with its claim to scientific verifiability within the limits of deterministic material-biochemical modes of action, appears rather backward in comparison.

It should be noted here, however, that modern physics and recent developments in medicine are gaining insights that seem to coincide with the millennia-old Far Eastern wisdom. For example, the topic of mind and matter discussed in the third chapter - an area of extraordinary importance for the healing arts of Ayurveda - is increasingly becoming the focus of modern medicine.

A close juxtaposition of these complex relationships, which were recognized long ago, should therefore be briefly pointed out to a better understanding of the old knowledge and to dispel possible prejudices.

I would point out to the reader that the following statements regarding cosmological views may seem too abstract and incomprehensible. If this is the case, I recommend that he or she skip these remarks and read on from the next subtitle.

I now begin this chapter with a (short) description from Krishna in the Bhagavadgita[19] of the immensity of the universe.

Krishna says, "I am in all hearts. I live everywhere in the cosmos as consciousness. Try to visualize the immensity and dizzying impermanence of the entire material universe, Arjuna - then you just start to get an idea of my absolute consistency. As you meditate on the total immensity of the cosmos, you begin to sense faint signs of the incomprehensible magnitude of my omnipresence."

Now let's take a look at the spiritual perspective of the Occident. Just a few centuries ago, ideas of religion and science in the Western Hemisphere were narrowed down in temporal and spatial dimensions!

Less than four hundred years ago, religious authorities and scientists, e.g. Bishop J. Usher, maintained that "our" planet was born on October 23, 4004 BC at 9 o'clock. In the seventeenth century, all scholars in the Occident – both spiritual and secular – calculated in these small temporal and spatial dimensions.

And today? The popular "Big Bang Theory" relocates the world's creation to about 13.7 billion years before our era. This still seems to be calculated in small temporal and spatial dimensions when one accounts for such considerations as the current loop quantum cosmology, which tries to explain what happened before the big bang.

A further development of loop quantum cosmology leads to a model of a cyclic universe, which always expands alternately to a maximum extent and then collapses.

It is amazing that this world view – we tend to say "a thought game" – was present several thousand years ago in the spirit of the Hindus.

A Brahma or Lord of Creation lives a hundred Brahma years. Each year consists of 360 Brahma days and a Brahma Day (Kalpa) holds 4,320,000,000 human years. [20] A Brahma day is followed by an equally long Brahma night. Thus, a complete world cycle takes 4,320,000,000 × 2 × 360 × 100 = 311,040 billion human years. This is followed by further corresponding cycles.

This may seem like a "utopian thought experiment" for "normal" minds, because, adjusted to the big bang theory, this temporal span seems unbelievable.

While it may be convenient to view this statement as inconsistent with modern scientific knowledge, it seems reasonable to suggest, by presenting these gigantic dimensions, a scale of meaning to demonstrate the immeasurable greatness of the gods, while the individual disappears into a "temporal nothingness."

However, man attains significance by participating in the incessant juxtaposition of creative and destructive cycles through rebirths, from which he can free himself if he develops spiritually.

This immense interplay of gigantic cycles conveys the message of the power of renewal and the transience of the existing.

Past, present and future co-exist in the absolute. I repeat Krishna in the Bhagavad Gita: "Try to visualize the tremendous vastness and dizzying inconstancy of the entire material universe, Arjuna - then you just start to get an idea of my absolute consistency."

In other words, the constant is the dizzying impermanence. The metaphor "everything flows" (πάντα ῥεῖ), ascribed to the Greek philosopher Heraclitus, also expresses that being cannot be understood statically but dynamically as eternal change.

Behind and at the same time in the incessant flow is unity, unity in multiplicity and multiplicity in unity.

The existence of eternal change is also expressed by Johann Wolfgang von Goethe in his poem "One and All".

From this, let me quote a passage. [21]
"Only moments seemingly stand still
The eternal excites in all
Because everything has to disintegrate into nothing
If it wants to insist in being"

These remarks indicate that the worldview of immense ages is not merely a "mind-game," but is a profound thought that captures immeasurable times and spaces that today also occupies modern physics.

Only about four hundred years ago did the dogma of a geocentric world order hesitantly give way to the recognition of a heliocentric view of the world, which however, is still incomplete.

On March 13, 1781 Herschel discovered the planet Uranus with a self-made reflector telescope in a systematic survey of the sky. With this discovery, the size of the solar system had doubled. With the discovery of the planet Neptune on September 23, 1846, the expansion of the solar system, ending so far at Uranus, had again almost been doubled in space!

Since then, the findings of these extended temporal and spatial dimensions have progressed more and more. The extent of the solar system is given today as three light years.

As an illustration it should be mentioned that one light year equals the distance that light travels at a velocity of nearly 300,000 km / sec. in a year, which is about 9.5 trillion kilometers.

The sun of "our" solar system is but a star of one hundred billion stars of "our" Milky Way, which extends in the plane over one hundred thousand light-years.

About forty neighboring galaxies make up the "Local Group" and one thousand three hundred to two thousand galaxies form the "Virgo Galaxy Cluster". Up to two hundred of these galaxy clusters in turn form the "Virgo Supercluster".

This is not the end of our contemplation of the immensity of the universe. Four years ago, a research team from the University of Hawai described the super galaxy cluster "Laniakea (immense sky) with an extension of five hundred twenty million light years and about one hundred thousand galaxies, including "our" Milky Way.

The newly found structure moves the Virgo Supercluster, formerly considered the Local Supercluster, to the rank of a mere part of Laniakea. In addition to Laniakea there are more super galaxy clusters including the Horologium supercluster with an extension of five hundred and fifty million light years.

A certain convergence between the recently acquired cosmic understanding of modern science of the Occident and the astonishingly conception of the Orient is illustrated here.

The question arises: are there in addition to the different views on cosmological contexts any similar discrepancies in other fields, such as medicine?

In this vast, incomprehensible background, man really seems to be comparable to a tiny cosmic speck of dust.

Professor K. V. Dilipkumar of Varier Ayurveda College, Kottakal, Kerala, sees here a misunderstanding that he attributes to a lack of true relationship to the universe [21a]. The idea of being like a pebble on the far bank, unlike other pebbles, is the misunderstanding.

Rather, man is part of a living organism that exists and works for the good of the organism, and that organism is the universe.

Apart from this consideration, however, an atom is more than nothing, as its nuclear fission and the associated release of enormous energy may make clear.

The subatomic world, in addition to the dizzying size of the macrocosm, opens up a dizzying immensity of the microcosm.

Thus – especially in recent decades, molecular biology – has caused a stir. In 1962, Francis Crick and James D. Watson received the Nobel Prize for Medicine in recognition of the decryption of the double helix structure of DNA molecules, the chemical compound that is the genetic material of all organisms.

Although the human genome has been officially decrypted since 2003, the significance of all genes is not yet known.

Worth mentioning here is that the international research project "Human Genome Project" could not confirm the thesis of "genetic determinism", but - as Martin G. Weiß in "The Dissolution of Human Nature".[22] explains – they came to the realization that there is no causal relationship between genotype and trait.

The expression of phenotypic features is rather a highly complex process of interactions and feedback between DNA, RNA, proteins and cytoplasm.

So it would make sense to see humans not merely as a "cosmic speck of dust" in which at best bio-chemical organic processes take place according to a predetermined pattern, but as a highly developed spiritual being in an extremely complex relationship of interactions and feedback, both with his inner world and the outer world.

Basic concepts: Vedanta and Sāṃkhya philosophy related to Ayurveda and Yoga

In the following, I briefly explain the Vedanta and Sāṃkhya philosophy (also written: Sānkhya), since some knowledge of these philosophical approaches is considered necessary for understanding the statements in this book.

Advaita Vedanta:

In Advaita Vedanta, the world is traced back to a single principle in a monistic system. The Sanskrit word advaita means non-duality. Thus, in particular, the essential identity of Atman (the individual soul) and Brahman (the world soul) is the core idea.

Shankara (c. 788-820 AD), one of the greatest scholars of Advaita Vedanta, described Brahman, the world soul, as having no form and attributes (nirguna).

Pure being (sat), pure consciousness (cit) and pure bliss (ananda) constitute the essence of Brahman, which are not to be understood as qualifying attributes.

In connection with Yoga, the "sister discipline" of Ayurveda, man can approach truth by various practices, i.e. recognizing the illusion (maya) through meditation, thus eliminating the ignorance (avidya) and therefore freeing the self from the non-self, attaining salvation (moksha).

In the dualistic system of Sāṃkhya philosophy, among others, the trigunas sattva, rajas and tamas are of importance. Thus, the ayurvedic medical system relies heavily on these three mental constitutions, as will be explained later.

In the Bhagavad Gita, the sacred book of the Hindus, both directions are addressed. Older texts suggest that Sāṃkhya presupposed a universal mind as the point of departure of the multiplicity. So it is understandable that in the Bhagavadgita and other texts Vedanta and Sāṃkhya are equally positioned without contradiction.

In addition to the Advaita-Vedanta there are modified directions such as Vishishtadvaita-Vedanta (qualified non-dualism), the Dvaitadvaita school (teaching simultaneous unity and difference), Dvaita-Vedanta (vedanta of duality: Atman and Brahman are eternally separated). In addition, other directions have emerged, which – in order not to go beyond the scope of the book – should not be addressed here.

Sāṃkhya (also Sāṅkhya):

Since Ayurveda's medical system is essentially based on the philosophical system of Sāṃkhya, a succinct explanation is given with a brief emphasis on some important factors of existence.

Sāṃkhya, one of the oldest philosophical schools of thoughts from Indian origin, basically represents a dualism within the framework of its metaphysics.

World events are traced back to two fundamental principles that shape the reality-determining elements of the world:

1. The passive, purely spiritual immutable soul, conscious mind (Purusha) and
2. The active, unconscious "primordial matter" or "nature" (Prakriti).

Krishna explains to Arjuna in the Bhagavadgita (chapters 7, 4-5) the two aspects of his divinity - a lower and a higher self.

The lower self is the realm of nature (Prakriti), consisting of the five elements, mind (Manas), intellect (Buddhi) and ego-consciousness (Ahamkara), the basic feeling of being in physical form.

Beyond the world of nature and different from nature, however, exists the spiritual aspect Purusha, the life force, the source of consciousness, the "soulfulness" of all life, which interacts with nature.

Purusha and Prakriti are without beginning (anadi) and infinite (ananta). In the original state there is no distinction between the two.

From Prakriti, all other factors of existence (tattvas) are to emerge in a process of "unfolding". Together with the Purusha and the Prakriti there is an enumeration of twenty-five Tattvas, from which the process of shaping the world is explained. Purusha is the self that is inherent in all sentient beings. It gives people, animals, plants and gods sensibility and awareness.

Thus also the Upanishads [23] describe an order of world principles, whose starting point is all that exists in Purusha to which the "unopened" is subordinate to the Avyakta (not yet manifested primary matter). This is followed by the Spirit manifesting in the world, the Great Self (Mahan Atman) and the subtle-minded higher cognitive faculty "Buddhi".

The Sanskrit word buddhi is derived from the root word buddh (awakening). Buddha is "the awakened," who achieves the purity and perfection of his mind through his own power, thus attaining a limitless unfolding of all the potentials in him, such as perfect wisdom "Prajna," and infinite-yet distant-compassion "Karuna" with all living things.

Buddhi refers to a transpersonal mental faculty of the mind, an "intuitive intelligence", more far-reaching than the rational mind.

Subordinate to Buddhi, the lower cognitive faculties "Manas" and finally the sensory organs "Indriya" follow.

In the Shvetashvatara Upanishad, "Ahamkara" (ego-maker or ego) - the objectively imagined consciousness of the individual, who refers to himself and understands himself as a single being - is classified between buddhi and manas.

Prakriti is the creative force behind all psycho-physical as well as material conditions of being, which also include physicality, thought processes and perception.

Ayurveda and Yoga:

Ayurveda and Yoga come as interconnected systems of Vedic knowledge, which describe the entire human life and the entire universe. A profound understanding of Ayurveda and Yoga in their original relationship to the sacred doctrine of the Vedas presupposes an awareness of this knowledge of Hinduism, first transmitted orally and later included in religious textbooks.

This cannot be taught in this book, due to its extremely extensive area. However, some core ideas are listed below and in the final chapter the magical connection of the "sister disciplines" Ayurveda and Yoga is explained in more detail.

Ayurveda:

The origin of Ayurveda as an essential aspect of Indian philosophy goes back over five thousand years, thus much earlier than the generally accepted birth of the history of philosophy in ancient Greece.

Gregory Bassham, Professor of Philosophy at Kings College, Pennsylvania, points out in this connection, in "250 Milestones in the History of Philosophy" [24], that in most of the standard works on the history of philosophy of Occidental authors philosophy begins with the ancient Greeks. He adds that, according to the American philosopher and historian Will Durant, the Indians and Chinese smile at this provincialism.

The religious and sacred ideas, the so-called Vedas, which were first transmitted orally, were later recorded in writing in four collections - Rigveda, Samaveda, Yajurveda and Atharva Veda. Ayurveda is a part of the Atharva Veda.

Ayurveda is the Vedic system, which promotes preventive measures, such as proper nutrition and a healthy lifestyle, and corrects an established imbalance in case of illness with holistic healing measures.

The origin of Ayurveda as medicine can be traced back approximately to the middle of the 2nd Millennium BC in the Vedic period. As a medical system, Ayurveda develops mainly from the Atharva Veda.

More than two thousand years ago, the Indian physician Caraka wrote a comprehensive compendium of ayurvedic medicine – the Caraka Samhita – which is still considered in modern times as an indispensable textbook for the study of Ayurveda.

Together with Suśrutasaṃhitā, a compendium on medicine and surgery written by the Indian surgeon Suśruta, these basic texts are the oldest ayurvedic works that have survived to this day and form the foundation of Ayurveda as a medical science.

Ayurveda is the first systematic collection of human knowledge. Through experience and constant experimentation, this continues to evolve to this day. Ayurveda has always seen man as a whole in his environment. Ayurveda, as a holistic medical system, addresses every element and every aspect of human life that is understood as part of the cosmic order. Ayurveda involves the insight that the universe as a macrocosm and man are directly related, reflect each other, and that each is present in the other.

This profound knowledge of human circumstances, has developed over thousands of years and forms the basis of the ayurvedic healing system. The inclusion of external factors such as climate, seasons, environmental conditions, diet, etc., allows the transfer of ayurvedic principles to the living conditions of humans.

Ayurvedic holistic medicine regards man as an individual, as a unity of body that is changeable, that is transient, of mind and soul, that is immutable, that is eternal.

First and foremost, Ayurveda is designed to be preventive, to maintain and improve physical, mental and spiritual health, to increase the vitality of the organism in order to achieve a state of happiness, harmony and contentment in all areas of life.

Diseases are not considered in isolation but are perceived as expressing a disturbed harmony between body, mind, soul and external factors.

Basic principle of the treatment is: The out of balance organism must be brought back into harmony. The holistic approach therefore takes into account the individual physical and mental constitution of the person concerned and does not "treat" a disease, but the human being, because the actual healing happens in the patient and by the patient.

The therapeutic measures are intended to support the physician's ability and desire to heal the patient. The therapy must be geared to the natural course of the disease for a certain period of time. If, however, the natural processes are ignored, this can weaken the natural healing powers.

This insight is also expressed in the statement "Medicus curat, natura sanat" (The doctor treats, nature heals), attributed to the Greek physician Hippocrates from Kos.

The version extended in the Christian Middle Ages by "Deus salvat" (God saves) points to the interaction of the physical, mental and spiritual and corresponds largely with the millennia-old knowledge of Ayurveda.

What is meant by the self-healing powers will be explained later. Before that, for a better understanding, some of the most important basic yoga concepts are described below.

Yoga

Yoga is the Vedic system which, in particular, addresses the spiritual sphere and, through spiritual practice, reverses the problems that may arise from suffered conditioning, such as mental block by reuniting the mind with pure consciousness.

The relationship of mind and body has been a particular problem in European intellectual history since antiquity, expressed in the concept of a separation of mind and body (dualism).

The philosophical traditions in Asia, on the other hand, are fundamentally based on a metaphysical assumption that sees this separation as an illusionary idea.

In an earlier publication[25] I have referred to something in this connection, which I will mention again in the next three paragraphs. Current paradigms of traditional science including biology are essentially based on three theses:
1. All material processes are due to atomic elementary processes
2. Consciousness and memory are only epiphenomena of nerve processes
3. The perception of an ego is based on a self-deception.

This (extreme) reductionism ascribes full reality to basic elements and not to the structures built from them.

This also seems to be consistent with the idea of the father of modern materialism by Thomas Hobbes. Only bodies can move and be moved only by the body. Also, processes of consciousness are understood only as a consequence of the movement of bodies (movements coming from the outside). Everything is determined there is no freedom of the will. All that is spiritual, as Epicurus assumed, is either a phantom or an illusion of matter in a highly refined form.

Similarly, in his causal dualistic worldview, Rene Descartes formulates a course within the object world. The human mind is a thinking thing (res cogitans) unlike bodies as extended things (res extensa). Two different substances, spirit and matter, interact and differ from the natural philosophy of Isaac Newton, according to which active immaterial "forces of nature" act on the absolutely passive matter.

Nobel laureate Erwin Schrödinger, one of the most significant scientists of the 20th century, points to the thesis of materialism, [26] that the mind is something material and replies: "such a position has the fundamental problem that the mind has properties which have no material object. Materialism must therefore explain how it may be that a material object has these qualities."

The idea of an immutable essence is unacceptable to most of today's philosophers because of their basic materialistic beliefs.

In "Science and Humanism: Physics in our Time," [27] Schrödinger addresses some of the most fundamental questions of the century:

How important is scientific research? And how do the achievements of modern science affect the relationship between material and spiritual things?

A key message is given here "It seems clear and obvious, but it must be said that the isolated knowledge acquired by a group of specialists in a narrow field has no intrinsic value, but only in its synthesis with all the rest of the knowledge and only insofar as it really contributes to answering the question in this synthesis, "Who are we?" You may ask - you must now ask me: What do you think is the value of science? I answer: Its scope, purpose and value are the same as any other area of human knowledge. No, none of them alone, only the union of all of them, has some scope or value at all, and that is simply enough described: It is to obey the command of the Delphic deity: gnothi seauton. (Know thyself).

In Chapter 3, I'll go into more detail about this "command".

According to Aurobindo, [28] the soul (the psychic being) stands behind the personality of man and has the ability to transform the nature of a person.

The psychic being can even protect the body from diseases and dangers. The psychic influences the consciousness from the background, but one has to step out of ordinary consciousness into the innermost being (psychic transformation) to find it, and one has to make it the ruler over the consciousness that it must be. Doing that is one of the main goals of yoga. [29]

The psychic being knows the way to the divine, hears its call and is able to lead the mind, heart and body to it. This must be done in a constant process until the contact with the Divine is stable and the Spiritual Transformation begins.

Once man has broken through the limitation of the mind, he looks at infinity, feels the eternal presence, an infinity of consciousness and bliss, a boundless self, an eternal divinity.

Further insights are given in the concluding chapter "Ayurveda and Yoga - the magic connection".

Physical constitution and mental constitution

Doshas (physical constitution) as well as Gunas (mental constitution) form the total wealth of the human constitution, but are also related to the total abundance of the world surrounding humans (cosmic principles).

Physical constitution

Of particular importance in Ayurveda are the gross physical elements and other determinants within the twenty-five Tattvas. The elements – called Mahabhutas – are the following:
Ākāśa (ether, space),
Vāyu (wind, air),
Tejas (fire, embers),
Jalam (water)
Pṛthivī (earth)

Note the hierarchy increasing from coarse density to lesser density elements and finally to the most subtle manifestation of Ākāśa.

The first four elements are also mentioned by Hippocrates and assigned to certain human characteristics, such as phlegmatic and earth, melancholic and water, choleric and fire and sanguine and air.

The fifth element Akāśa is unknown to Hippocrates.
Ayurveda, on the other hand, does not assign human characteristics to only one element, but to a certain mixture, such as kapha with earth and water, pitta with fire and water, and vata with air and ether.

Ayurvedic medicine is based in the core on the three fundamental governing forces or bio-energies, the three Dohas (Vata, Pitta and Kapha), which are related to the five elements of earth, water, fire, air and ether.

These are responsible for the anatomical and physiological activities in the body. Their harmony with each other is crucial for a person's health. If there is a disturbance of the Dosha ratio, this is called Vikriti.

The physical constitution defined at conception is composed of a certain ratio of mix and determines certain framework conditions for the entire lifespan of the respective human being, which will be explained later.

Some of the Tattvas are briefly mentioned here, which later in the book are explained in more detail: Buddhi is intelligence, cognition, Ahamkara is the ego consciousness (ego), Manas means reason based thinking.

Sāṃkhya had a close connection with yoga early on. Sāṃkhya provided the theory and yoga the practice.
    Due to this complementary aspect, the two systems are also known under the combination of words "Sāṃkhya-Yoga".

From the beginning – as the ayurvedic teachings say – the world consists of five elements: space (or ether), air, fire, water and earth.

They determine everything: the essence of stones, plants, animals and humans. All elements are also found in the human body, for example in the five senses: listening (space), seeing (fire), smelling (earth), feeling (air) and tasting (water).

Since the different elements are pronounced in every human being at birth – actually already at conception –to varying degrees, Ayurveda starts from a complex human individuality. Each and every one is endowed with particular physical and emotional strengths and weaknesses. To which type a person can be counted is determined by the mixing ratio of the three doshas (Vata, Pitta and Kapha), which in turn are composed of the five elements.

These three main doshas are well known. Less popular, however, are the five associated subdoshas, which interact with each other and influence the energetic dynamics in the organism. [30]

Therefore, the most important relationships are briefly explained here.

The five subdoshas of Vata are conceived as parts of the life breath, as life energy of nature.

Impairments of Vata are usually based on disorders of the subdoshas:

1. Prana as a propulsive breath enables the mental and emotional sensory experiences
2. Udana is the rising breath and allows speaking, breathing, swallowing
3. Samana as the absorbing breath allows the digestion, assimilation of nutrients
4. Apana as down-directed breath allows excretion. Apana is also referred to as the root of Vata. If Apana is disturbed, it usually shows up in the holding of negative thoughts and feelings and in the lack of ability to let go.
5. Vyana as outflowing breath is responsible for the circulation, nervous system and sense of touch.

Symptoms of a Vata disorder– mostly caused by grief, worry, excitement, too much raw food, excessive sports – include anxiety, restlessness, constipation, lack of concentration, insomnia, hypersensitivity, inner restlessness.

If there are impairments, for example in the form of gastrointestinal disturbances, bladder weakness, weak nerves, or sleeping disorders, a gentle abdominal massage with sesame oil heated to body temperature will relieve the symptoms, when applied in the evening before bed.

The five subdoshas of Pitta are characterized by the following causal relationships:

1. Pacaca regulates primary digestion
2. Ranjaka controls the secondary digestion and blood formation
3. Sadhaka influences intelligence and knowledge
4. Alocaca governing vision
5. Bhrajaka has an effect on skin color, body temperature

The references explain the properties of Pitta, which physiologically relate to the metabolism, especially on the digestion and heat balance, intellect and emotion.

Disturbed Pitta can be compensated by appropriate nutrition. Recommended foods include:
asparagus, zucchini, peas, broccoli, potatoes, savoy cabbage, lettuce, basmati rice, milk (not homogenized), cottage cheese, green beans, fresh peas, sunflower oil, coconut oil, mangoes, sweet melons, avocado, pears, figs, pineapple, apples, coriander, cinnamon, turmeric, ginger, sunflower and pumpkin seeds.

The characteristics of the subdoshas of Kapha are the following:
1. Bodhaka, associated with water, allows in the form of saliva in the mouth the taste and the liquefaction of the food.
2. Kledaka is responsible for the first stage of digestion in the stomach.
3. Avalambaka corresponds to the plasma in the body – the primary water element – is distributed in the body through the lungs and heart activity.
4. Tarpaka is associated with the cerebrospinal fluid in the brain, which is crucial for contentment, emotional balance, and good memory.
5. The practice of yoga also enhances the mental form of Kapha as contentment and bliss (Ananda).
6. Shleshaka corresponds to the synovial fluid, the quality of water that gives lubrication. It is responsible for keeping the joints together.

People who are predominantly Kapha tend to swamp quickly. Light diet to promote the digestive fire is recommended. Sweet and fatty food should be limited. To promote the digestive juices it is recommended to enhance the dishes with ginger, black pepper, coriander, turmeric, cloves, cardamom.

It is crucial in Ayurveda that the human body is seen not merely as a material body in which bio-chemical processes take place, but as "ayur" as a living unity of body, mind and soul.

Man is soul and mind is stronger than genes. [31]

With this key statement, cell biologist Bruce Lipton, along with others, dispels the traditional dogma that man is a prisoner of his genetic heritage. We are not victims who have to take over the sufferings of our ancestors fatefully.

The personal life of a person as well as the collective existence is determined primarily by interactions between mind and matter and less controlled by the DNA. [32]

Mind and matter correspond. Energy and information fields determine physiology and biochemistry. Thinking and feeling as well as the perception of the environment works into every cell, controls genes and determines life.

Mental constitution

According to Sāṃkhya, the ethereal basic components of creation (Prakrti) are characterized by three essential properties (Gunas), which are harmoniously combined in their original state.

Ethereal is understood in this context as an immaterial property. The trigunas are:

Tamas (laziness, darkness, heaviness, chaos),

Rajas (restlessness, movement, energy) and

Sattva (being, clarity, harmony, purity).

Swami Sivananda [33] comments on the Gunas as those are mentioned in the Bhagavad Gita:

As the sun illuminates the day, Sattva awakens knowledge and enlightens intellect.

By contrast, insatiable desire and blindness to the interests and feelings of others are the negative aspects of Raja and stupor and ignorance the negative aspects of Tama.

The nature of man is shaped by his virtues and mistakes, whereby the overall picture and not one or two characteristics of the Gunas is determinative.

These cosmic principles can be developed and sublimated in man as mental constitutions.

Spiritual development is of particular importance to health.

Man consists mainly of the earth and water element. The earth element is the densest and heaviest of the five elements and contains the highest proportion of Tama, an expansion-limiting component.

Through spiritual practice, the relationship of the ethereal components can be changed in favor of sattva and existence can be extended until finally expectations and desires disappear and one rests in the real self (Swasthya) and is perfectly happy. Such mentally-developed people radiate a noticeable charisma. These relationships are of particular importance in Ayurveda as well as in Yoga, as will be shown later.

2. Modern medicine without soul?

"I dissected a lot of bodies, but I did not find a soul." This remark – with which he wanted to say that there is no soul – is attributed to the famous Privy Councilor Rudolf Virchow, the founder of cellular pathology.

It could be argued that the search for a soul in the lifeless body is from the outset a doomed undertaking.

And further, Virchow stated amongst other findings: [34]:
"That's what I call anatomical thought in medicine. I assert that no doctor is able to properly think about a pathological process when he is unable to direct to its place in the body. Ubi est morbus is the question. Research on sedes morbi has progressed from organs to tissues, from tissues to cells. But at the same time practical medicine has extended the principle of local treatment more and more, and, in a still unimaginable extent, has applied it even to innermost parts of the body, which until then were regarded as completely unapproachable. Both pharmacology and surgery have become more focused on a specific part of the body each year".
Here the very different view is expressed, namely that of a locally determined fixed point of the "sedes morbus" as an indispensable condition for the assignment of a pathological process, and the holistic view of Ayurveda, which understands man as a whole being in his environment.

To be able to successfully treat, the answer to the question "where is the seat of the disease" is certainly a first prerequisite. But often the search for a weak spot in the body, which favors the development of a disease (locus minoris resistentiae), however, has led to it and still leads today to symptomatic treatment, rather than to search for where the cause lies.

Exactly one hundred years later, Nobel laureate, molecular biologist and neuroscientist Francis H.C. Crick formulates in his book "What the soul really is" [35]: "You, your joys and sorrows, your memories and ambitions, your sense of one's identity and free will, all of this, in fact, is just the behavior of a huge collection of nerve cells and related molecules." Thus, about twenty-four years ago, Crick believed that he had demystified the soul and placed it on a natural scientific foundation.

Louis Cozolino, a clinically practicing psychologist, sees the self, localized in a particular brain region [36] and assumes that the self consists of many layers of neuronal processing that develop from bottom to top during growth.

Karl Wimmer[37] refers to Gerhard Roth, one of the leading brain researchers, who clearly described Crick's approach as too reductionist. "Crick does not go into the big difference between soul, mind and consciousness at all. He is ultimately looking for consciousness neurons, i.e. those nerve cells that raise awareness through their activity. The blatant weakness of such reductionism is that there is absolutely nothing spiritual or cognitive about the activity of a single neuron." [38]

Like Crick's remarks, the findings of Cozolino suggest that "the insula and the anterior cingulate cortex may be involved in the early development and ongoing organization of the self".

Here, too – as was concluded earlier in Virchow's "search for the soul" – an attempt condemned to failure from the outset is recognizable, to interpret the soul as non-existent, or to define the self by focusing solely on the activity of nerve cells.

This does not, however, give the antithesis of the existence of a soul, of a possible existing in the unknown. "Absence of evidence is no evidence of absence". (Carl Sagan)

I will not continue to adhere to this consideration and analysis of the existence or nonexistence of the soul which has been practiced since ancient times, since I am not in a position to add anything essential and such an investigation would be too far reaching in the context of this book.

At this point, rather remarkable comments are inserted, for example, by the writer Stefan Zweig, which he formulated in 1931 – 37 years after the denial of the existence of a soul by Virchow – in "Healing by the Spirit" on this topic. It is also noteworthy that these remarks are still relevant today, ninety years later.

I quote [39]:"Modern medicine works with factual certainties instead of individual intuitions, and although it likes to poetically call itself > medical art<, this high word can only be applied in the limited sense of arts and crafts.

...Scientific medicine regards the patient and his illness as an object and almost dismissively assigns to him the role of absolute passivity; he has nothing to ask and nothing to say, nothing to do but to obey the orders of the doctor obediently and even thoughtlessly and to eliminate himself as far as possible from the treatment... whereas in scientific medicine the patient is "treated" as an object, spiritual healing requires the patient first of all to act emotionally, to develop the highest possible activity against the disease as the subject, carrier, and principal provider of the cure."

And further[40]: "Everything that is psychically irregular for the mechanistic conception of that time is merely a degeneration of the nerves, a pathological change; The impertinence prevails imperturbable, it can succeed thanks to an ever more accurate knowledge of the organs and with experiments from the animal kingdom to precisely calculate the automatic of the > mental <, to correct any deviation .... So Freud too has to first sit at the dissecting table with all kinds of technical equipment and look for causes which in truth never reveal in the gross form of sensual visibility."

An amazing insight of the writer!

Modern medicine likes to speak of a victory against one or another disease that are interpreted as enemies. Myriads of medicines are offered through a wide network of pharmacies to fight countless illnesses. Nevertheless, the so-called civilization diseases are constantly increasing. This has led to an immense build-up of defensive measures using state-of-the-art techniques for symptom analysis and complex treatment of illnesses, allowing the root causes to slip out of sight.

According to Virchow's dogma does modern medicine, as an apparatus medicine under the pressure of scientific measurable verifiability, pursue a medicine without soul, which at the same time gets caught up in a "fight against windmills" (symptom control)?

Mbih Jerome Tosam, Doctor of Philosophy at the University of Yaoundé, one of the largest universities in Cameroon, sees one of the weaknesses of modern Western medicine in its over-dependence on the Cartesian ontology (doctrine of being), which considers human bodies as machines. [41]

These must be studied with scientific logic.

Finally, when the physician, as a technician, has the task of repairing dysfunctional bodies, this modern perspective leads to neglect the patient as a subjective being.

This deficiency can only be remedied by overcoming the Cartesian reductionist worldview responsible for this.

For example, I consider it appropriate in the following to present some noteworthy comments, such as those that are critical of the trend of modern medicine, when only geared towards objectively scientifically verifiable evidence.

In particular, evidence-based medicine (EBM) – as currently practiced – is the focus of criticism.

Subsequently, recent developments in "classical medicine" are addressed, which overcome the just mentioned reductionist dogma. These findings have introduced a change in mainstream medicine in recent decades that is more open to holistic understanding.

Evidence Based Medicine (EBM) of Ayurveda and Medicine Based Evidence (MBE) of Modern Medicine

The surgeon Bernd Hontschik, for example sees a danger in the trend of modern medicine using guidelines of evidence-based medicine (EBM) to focus only on objectively existing reality that alone it is to recognize.

This is that "guidelines act as a leveling off of the subjective, thereby putting both the practitioner and the patient in danger of losing an essential element of vitality".[42]

Hontschik affirms that medical art consists in treating the sick as a subject, as a living being.

Another problem is the misconception that modern knowledge supposedly already means science.

Dr. Remya Krishnan, a significant Ayurvedic personality and Associate Professor of Rajiv Gandhi Ayurveda Medical College, Government of Puducherry, sees in the Western medical approach – as currently practiced and frequently updated (EBM) – nothing but medicine-based evidence (MBE). [43]

In other words, evidence is defined by statistical methods and not really linked to fundamental science.

Dr. R Krishnan concludes that "integration of presently Western-based MBE in evidence-based Ayurveda is ineffective in achieving good health and well-being. Modern medicine makes use of drugs that act on both targeted and non-targeted tissues through abnormal stimulation and cause suppression of the immune system (blocking the immune response).

Ayurveda relies on findings from guideline principles of fundamental science that ensure the safety and efficacy of applied medicine.

In Ayurveda, it is not just the diagnosis of disease itself that is so important but rather the identification of the responsible complex etiological factors and their deep interconnectedness, which are the real causes and derive the consequent effects.

Modern medicine is not familiar with this kind of profoundly functional knowledge; rather, it is involved with intensive differentiation to every system of the human body. Super-specialists who have trained in modern medicine know a lot of rather limited branches of medicine, but little in terms of the central regulatory processes of functional coordination between the various organ systems in the body."

Relying on the claim to be scientific and the willingness to support the general acceptance of Ayurveda in Western culture, various agencies endeavor to integrate Ayurveda into conventional medicine. This undertaking fails to recognize that today's medicine, with its claim to scientific knowledge, still uses a science of the nineteenth century and de facto develops into an appendage of the pharmaceutical industry and a profitable health system. [44]/[45]

At this point I refer to Issac Matthai, ayurvedic chief physician of Soukhya, the holistic center in Bengaluru, who emphasizes [46] "in order to achieve truly profound healing, the patient must consciously make a shift on the mental and emotional level and rebuild the perception of the self (Swasthya).

Only then can a real state of balance be restored to body-mind-soul. Drugs do not heal, they only control or suppress symptoms. Western medical models tend to ignore the cause of the disease because its focus is elsewhere and de facto become an appendage to the pharmaceutical industry and profitable health care.

I hope that understanding health care in the future will not be primarily about treating and curing diseases, but about maintaining health and preventing disease."

The inseparable connectedness of body, mind and soul of the mesocosm human is a basic concept of Ayurveda.

"The awareness of the soul is the deepest healing process ever, not only for the soul, but also for the mind.

The perception of the soul releases all healing powers." [47]

Subsequent words of Jiddu Krishnamurti may reveal the limitations of human thought and encourage further reflection:

"The human mind that exists in the realm of the known can never invite the unknown". [48]

Psychosomatic medicine

It is noteworthy that, for example, the psychosomatic approach today still applies to a medical system that corresponds in many areas to the causality principle of the mechanistic Cartesian world view and seeks to associate a disease with a particular (monocausal) specific cause. [49]

In addition, the term "psychosomatic" is often equated by laymen as well as medical professionals with "psychogenic". As a result, patients suffering from physical symptoms often feel misunderstood as imaginary patients.

The word composition originating from the Greek language stands for a combination of soul and body. "Psychosomatic means that body and soul are two inseparable aspects of human beings that are distinguished only for methodological reasons or for better understanding." [50]

However, there is no such thing as "linear" causality in the sense that mental disorders cause physical illnesses and thus diseases exist with mental origin and diseases with somatic causes.

"Mental problems do not cause physical disorders: They are!" [51]

A shift in the field of psychosomatic medicine has been initiated, inter alia, by Thure von Uexküll in the 1960s - when Crick was at the height of his research and deciphering DNA.

Immediately after his appointment to the University of Ulm in the Department of Internal Medicine and Psychosomatic Medicine in 1966, Thure von Uexküll initiated a reform of medical studies through the integration of subjects such as psychology and sociology.

In 1992, he founded the Academy of Integrated Medicine with the aim of bringing back the psychosocial dimension lost in Western culture to all fields of medicine.

He lamented the "dualistic paradigm" of medicine with the division into a "sick body without soul and a suffering soul without body." He had the idea of an "integrated medicine" that overcomes the prevailing biomechanical / psychological dualism in medical care.

In addition to the observations on psychosomatics, a significant connection with the placebo and nocebo effect is explained, followed by some comments on the relationship and mechanisms of action of psycho-neuro-endocrine socio-immunology.

Placebo and Nocebo

Mock treatments with drugs that do not contain an effective drug and thus have no pharmacological effect caused by such a substance, but are based on a psychosocial context of treatment, have been known as placebo phenomena in medicine for decades and extensively studied.

The word placebo comes from Latin and means "I will please".

The 1985 Nobel Peace Prize laureate and cardiologist Bernard Lown, describes in his book The Lost Art of Healing [52], how medical communication and patient expectations have both significant positive and negative effects on the course of medical treatment.

"Words are the most powerful tool a doctor has. Words, however, can - like a double-edged sword - hurt and heal."

The power of a medical's words or of another medical practitioner leads to healing or injury, and is characterized by the authority and certainty with which information is conveyed and, "above all else, by the willingness to listen to the patient".
It is the power of being together with others that forms and shapes our brain. [53]

With the discovery of endorphins ("happiness hormones") in the late 1970s, it was shown that placebos can be used to release endorphins, among other things, and to eliminate pain receptors.

The Nocebo phenomenon, which is the counterpart of the placebo phenomenon, has come into the focus of basic science and clinical medicine only in recent years. Nocebo means "I will hurt".

According to Lown, a careless word or unjustified pessimism can lead the patient into depression, delay healing, or even speed their death.

He describes a case in which he once witnessed how a surgeon, after opening the abdomen of a cancer patient, told the patient that the cancer had spread everywhere and further effort would be in vain. As a result, the patient died the same day. This incident reminds him of the so-called voodoo death, where a victim is given a certain spell and consequently dies within 24 hours. The panic a victim may experience after pronouncing a death spell is as deadly as a dose of poison.

It is still unclear for doctors and researchers how exactly the Nocebo phenomenon originates and which processes take place in the body.

Some explanations assume that the patient's expectation is important, for example, when administering a drug with regard to possible side effects, the patient expects the occurrence of this or that side effect.

This negative expectation lowers the level of endorphins in the blood and the deficit of these so-called happiness hormones leads to the damaging effect of the Nocebo. In addition, in the case of negative expectation, anxiety or panic, a hormone acting as a neurotransmitter in the brain releases the messenger substance cholecystokonin (CCK). The patient feels worse and more sensitive to pain, even if no pain receptors are irritated. [54]

Walter Feichtinger has investigated the nocebo effect and a series of theories in connection with the voodoo death [55] which shed some light on the interactions of psyche, nervous, hormonal and immune systems and which are therefore briefly discussed here.

According to one idea, the voodoo death is caused by overstimulation of the sympathetic-adrenal system in the absence of follow-up action. A counter opinion considers the hopelessness and the over activity of the parasympathetic nervous system as responsible for the sudden death.

Another theory is that both the sympathetic and the parasympathetic react accordingly to influences, such as active ingredients or even mental activity with "tuning". While one system reacts in a first phase, the other one is reduced.

As the stimulation increases further, eventually the other system is completely inhibited. In a second phase, the excited system also responds to stimuli that usually should address the antagonistic system.

With further stimulation, finally, the balance of both systems tilts completely and both work simultaneously. With increasing activation of the two linked systems, the ability to think logically decreases until a clear thinking is finally no longer possible.

It should be noted that obviously influencing factors – without scientific proof of a specific effect – can cause a positive or negative reaction.

Hope, which leads to an increase in social interaction and communication, apparently improves the physical constitution. Biopsychological effects are activated, hormone secretion, immune system, heart activity stimulated. In addition, a hopeful person can deal better with stress.

Fear and hopelessness, on the other hand, do exactly the opposite. "In extreme cases, hope can be expressed through miraculous self-healing and the hopelessness through voodoo death." [56]

The recognition of this psycho-neurological interdependence allows for a better understanding of the causative factors and provides approaches for causal treatment neglecting the obsolete symptomatic treatment.
    A recent interdisciplinary field of research explores these interactions in an expanded context and is known under the complex word structure of socio-psycho-neuro-endocrino-immunology.

This is briefly discussed below, as here important findings of modern medicine with ancient wisdom of Ayurveda and yoga cover, as will be explained later in more detail.

Socio-Psycho-Neuro-Endocrino-Immunology

The interacting cooperation between the immune system and the nervous system (psycho-neuro-immunology) and simultaneous learning ability was experimentally demonstrated by the American researcher Robert Ader in 1974, thus providing the impetus for research in one of the most important areas of modern medicine. [57]

By incorporating hormonal interactions and interactions of the social environment, this research area has been expanded to socio-psycho-neuro-endocrine immunology.

As already mentioned, the basis of this finding is the fact that messenger substances of the nervous system act on the immune system and messengers of the immune system on the nervous system. Interfaces of the control circuits are the brain with the pituitary gland, the adrenals and the immune cells. For example, neuropeptides have the property of docking to immune cells and affecting both the velocity and direction of movement of macrophages (cells of the immune system).

Through these connections it can be explained with the help of psychosomatics why psychological and psychotherapeutic processes have a demonstrable effect on bodily functions.

Of particular interest in research is the recognition of dependencies of the immune cells on the psyche, e.g. the question of why stress can negatively influence immune factors.

However, a variety of functions and interactions of immune cells is not fully understood.

Some negative or positive psychological factors influencing the immune defense[58] are presented below, in particular with regard to comparative knowledge of Ayurveda and Yoga, which are explained in more detail below.

Dependencies of the immune cells on the psyche

Negative mental factors have been shown to weaken the immune system, while positive psychic factors correlate with better functioning of the immune system.

Stress:
Stress occurs in different ways and can be perceived very differently.

Characteristics of the stressors are expressed in the duration of only short-lasting to chronic stress.

Furthermore, stressors located further back in time may have left traumas behind. The subjective feeling can be perceived as a challenge or overburdening, which one assumes one is unable to cope with.

Short-term stress (acute stress) can – as studies show – increase the nonspecific innate immune system (Eustress).

In chronic stress (Distress), both the innate and adaptive immune systems respond with immuno-suppression and other misconduct. [59]

In chronic stress, the increased secretion of glucocorticoids act as immuno-suppressants, as has been demonstrated. Furthermore, the activity of T- and B-lymphocytes is reduced in chronic stress.

T-lymphocytes are responsible for the so-called cellular immune response. The main task of B-lymphocytes is the formation of antibodies that circulate in the blood.

With the reduction of immune factors the frequency of infection increases. This can provoke the onset or worsening of disease. In this situation, termed "open window", the immune system can no longer adequately eliminate pathogens.

Depression:

Depression can also reduce the immune system. Scientifically recognized is a reduced activity of NK cells associated with the weakening of a major pillar of the immune system.

Natural killer cells (NK cells) belong to the lymphocytes and are part of innate immunity. The defense reaction of NK cells plays an important role in the early immune response and is directed against the body's own degenerate cells such as virus-infected cells and tumor cells.

Fear:

Regarding anxiety disorders, as well as stress and depression, different effects on the immune system could be demonstrated. For example, a reduction in lymphocyte production (adaptive immune system) could be consistently detected.

Further research is seeking to identify a more specific relationship between mental anxiety and functional changes in the immune system.

So much is mentioned here to the negative mental factors.

Positive psychological factors strengthen the immune system, as proven by various studies.

A positive attitude to life has been shown to increase the number of diverse cells involved in the immune system.

For example, feelings of gratitude, contentment, happiness and serenity not only have an effect on faster healing success after injury or surgery, but also have positive effects on the effectiveness and regulation of the immune system.

Optimism:

Optimists are generally happier people than pessimists. They are usually more self-confident and more balanced and see the often mentioned glass as half full rather than half empty. Optimists tend to assess the likelihood that something good will happen to them higher than the likelihood of a negative event happening to them.

On the one hand, although this "unrealistic optimism" contributes to well-being, it also carries the risk of underestimating dangerous situations.

Since in general positive consequences of an unrealistically high optimism outweigh the negative consequences, it obviously pays to see the glass half full. [60]

Worth noting here is that several studies prove that optimism reinforces the functions of the immune system.

For example, a slower course of disease in HIV-positive patients could be observed if they showed an optimistic attitude and conversely, a rapid deterioration of the overall condition was detectable when they had given up themselves.[61]

Social bonds:

Interpersonal relationships characterized by intense emotions correspond to an innate human need.

The certainty of receiving social recognition and support creates a sense of belonging and security.

Again, various studies have shown that social support from family and friends is associated with a good balance of some of the cells involved in the immune system.

In particular, it has been demonstrated that the number of NK cells has been significantly increased by the social support experienced. [62]

Social relationships – especially attachment relationships – not only build pleasant feelings between people, but also have a formative influence on the brain and can change the brain structure over the course of a lifetime, as explained below.

Now life experiences not only shape the brain, but leave an impression in the psyche and trigger off, depending on the negative or positive feelings, a corresponding reaction of the immune cells.

Interpersonal neurobiology - the social synapse

A synapse is the site of a neural connection through which a nerve cell is in contact with another cell.

Mutual communication between neurons occurs via chemical signals, with neurons interacting with each other through the transmission of biochemical messengers.

Comparatively, the clinical psychologist, psychotherapist, theologian and philosopher Louis Cozolino calls the transmission of communication between human brains a "social synapse". [63]

The social synapse is the interpersonal space and at the same time the medium in which larger organisms such as families, tribes, societies and the human species as a whole are communicatively integrated.

Just as individual neurons in the brain communicate with each other via synaptic transmission via chemical signals, communication between people, according to Cozolino, consists of the same "basic building blocks".

Interpersonal neurobiology assumes that the brain is a social organ whose structure is developed through life experiences. Already the experiences of the first years of life exert a high influence on the development of the brain and the formation of further nerve tissues.

The interaction of the nervous structure and experiences takes place through permanent feedback from the brain to social behavior and conversely from social behavior to the brain.

Interpersonal relationships – especially attachment relationships – have a formative influence on the brain and can alter the brain structure over the course of a lifetime. Thus, a negative environment exerts adverse effects on the brain structure, whereas harmonic associations have positive effects.

This connection was obviously no secret to Russian writer Leo Tolstoy a hundred and thirty years ago. He begins his novel and classic of world literature "Anna Karenina" with the sentence "All happy families are alike, every unhappy family is unhappy in their own way."

This formulation, which has become known as the "Anna Karenina Principle", cannot be limited to family psychology but also to other areas, such as economic life.

Humans influence each other's internal biological state and in the long run mutually influence the structure of the human brain.

Cozolino criticizes the Western science and philosophy and he accuses it of seeking answers that are technical and abstract "rather than looking for them in lived experiences and human interactions." [64]

"In neurobiology and neuroscience, researchers have examined the brain with scanners and on the dissecting table, but they have often neglected the fundamental context of social interaction in which the brain should flourish and thrive.

Nowhere is the struggle between paradigms more evident than in psychiatry with its dual history in psychoanalysis and neurology "

So man does not live isolated as an individual in his environment, but body, mind and soul are constantly experiencing a change in interacting with the social environment and nature as a prerequisite for life.

In order not to be at the mercy of feelings, one needs to recognize many influencing factors and a harmonious adaptation, in other words, becoming conscious and gaining self-knowledge.

3. Consciousness - know yourself

The following preface is intended to indicate the current labile - if not threatening - social lifestyle of the predominantly western hemisphere. At this point in the book, let the reader pay close attention to an increasing attitude to life of indifference and disinterest towards the social community which is more and more threatened.

Moral crisis

How does the individual want to keep healthy, mentally spiritually intact, if he lives in a society where numerous political leaders and their economic and financial magnates present a destructive life-concept through unscrupulous, corrupt, deceitful ways of life, in a society whose religious leaders are unable to counteract this activity with an effective spiritual counterforce?

Five hundred years ago, Niccolo Machiavelli described politics as the sum of the means necessary to come to power and hold on to power and to make the most useful use of power.

One could say "the end justifies the means". However, the prescription of the most useful use is reversed and misused to safeguard asocial self-interest.

Where does that lead? In the worst case, a reckless power politics taking advantage of all means. The abuse of power inevitably leads to moral crisis, if not to social collapse.

Matthias Weik concludes: "There is much to suggest that the moral crisis of our society is not a consequence of economic crashes, but that the decline of morality makes the crisis possible." [65]

It's not just about economic and fiscal system crises, it's about a major systemic crisis affecting social, moral and human factors.

C.G. Jung states a sense of helplessness among so many people in Western societies:

"They have begun to realize that our troubles are moral and we can not solve them by accumulating nuclear weapons or through economic competition. Many of us now understand that moral and mental remedies are more effective because they could make us immune to the ever-increasing infection." [66]

And further: "As our scientific understanding has increased, our world has become dehumanized.

Man feels isolated in the cosmos because he is no longer connected to nature and has lost his emotional unconscious identity with natural phenomena."

Back to Matthias Weik: "We cannot avoid asking the question of meaning at this point: What is the meaning of our existence?

Today we live alongside each other, instead of with each other. We are all part of the problem - we are all part of the solution!

What does this mean in relation to health policy?

Planning, organization, control and financing of the health system, negotiations with associations of health insurance companies, with doctors and pharmacists, with the pharmaceutical industry, together with regulation of corresponding laws and directives are one side of the coin.

Health in All Policies, on the other hand, appears more important and more effective for the health of the population by influencing other health-related areas of politics and life, such as education, work, housing, nutrition, transport, environment, family, leisure.

As Matthias Weik explains: "Through education, values, morality and ethics are conveyed, as well as self-evident humility and gratitude and respect for life and nature.

Only in this way can a natural, socially deeply rooted life grow free of greed and exaggerated selfishness ".

Spiritual development

What does Ayurveda contribute in this regard?

Can awareness, self-awareness, self-esteem be preventive of negative social attributes?

As already mentioned in the spiritual constitution (Gunas), man can influence his spiritual development.

Depending on the depth of his knowledge, he lives in lethargic form (Tamas), in living form (Rajas) or in self-confident form (Sattwa).

The person living in sloth is not or is only partially aware of the effects of his lifestyle. He does not question the consequences of his actions, he is exposed to the laws of nature and experiences various suffering.

The living person is aware of the dangers of the hallucinations and his actions. He strives to keep the consequences in moderation.

The self-conscious man rests in the self (Swasthya). He recognizes the forces and dangers inherent in him and resists temptations such as desires, value judgments and dogmas. He lives in reason (Buddhi), is a loving person, a reckless ego is alien to him.

This behavior says a lot. But what is this self in essence, what does self-knowledge mean for man?

The challenging inscription "Know thyself" (gnothi seauton) in the temple of Delphi is well known and is often quoted.

However, the second part of the message in the temple "so that you recognize the divine within you" is largely unknown and therefore remains unmentioned.

Here are three essential aspects addressed: the self, the knowledge and the divine in man. Since only the first part is popular it is not surprising that knowledge or self-knowledge is sought with knowledge on an intellectual level, without considering the divine aspect in this context.

What is addressed with the "divine in you"?

Most of the people I have encountered in my life and with whom I have spoken are afflicted with a kind of mental fear of contact – or at least an irritation – when talking about the "divine".

Again and again my interlocutors say that an "enlightened" person of modernity cannot do anything with the "divine". The motto of the Enlightenment "Sapere aude" (have courage to use your own mind) is to challenge your own mind and this will come to the realization that the so-called divine in mankind simply has faith-related religious significance.

Moreover, it is incompatible with the Christian faith to speak of the divine in man, since humans are not gods.

Well, the southern German "griaß di God" is familiar to us, with which the wish is expressed, God greet you, originally "may God bless you".

The Hindu and generally Indian greeting "Namaste" is not so common in Western culture, but quite popular among yoga practitioners in the West.

This greeting, rather casually applied in India, is carried out with a slight bow with hands in front of the chest near the heart with palms touching.

Namaste is a Sanskrit word that reveals several meanings when studying deeper. Literally translated it means. I lean in front of you (Nama is the bow). The most common meaning is "I bow to the divine in you" or "God in me bows to the God in you".

Again, this statement encounters opposition from the Christian faith, for Isaiah says there is only one God, and he does not share his glory. [67] The Old Testament states, "Thou shalt have no other gods beside me[68]. A bow or some kind of respect for another god is therefore idolatry.

Is there a conflict or is there a commonality?

In order to make a statement as a Christian concerning statements of another religion, one should first examine the meaning and source of this statement.

The following may contribute to this.

Aadil Palkhivala, considered to be one of the most recognized yoga teachers of the present, having studied Ayurveda intensively and having a professional degree in law, physics, and mathematics, as well as being author of "Fire of Love," interprets Namaste as "the belief in a divine spark which is found in every human being in the heart chakra.

The gesture is a recognition of the soul by the soul in another." [69]

Krishna teaches Arjuna in the Bhagavagita[70] the difference of divine knowledge (Jnana) and divine wisdom (Vijnana).

Recognition and knowledge are acquired through the senses, such as the sight and the mind.

Wisdom is attained through direct apprehension, insight and intuition.

Knowledge happens on a rational level, wisdom realizes the knowledge and is able to apply it in daily life. If both come together, there is nothing further that is worth knowing. [71]

Even though today it is generally acknowledged that knowledge is based primarily on meaningful understanding and wisdom on intuition, it is pointed out that modern man – initiated by secularization – no longer understands his origin in a divine creator.

The physicist and philosopher Fritjof Capra sees this as a loss of full humanity, marked by Cartesian anxiety, caused by the separation of mind and body. [72]

It would be possible to regain full humanity if the relationships of the cultural and social network of life surrounding mankind are recognized and if man experiences a re-coupling to this surrounding network of life.

Mata Satyamayi comments on the forty verses on the Self of Sri Ramana Maharshi [72a]:

Despite of all external influences of the Occident, the Indian mentality lacks the rupture that the Enlightenment (secularization) has brought into the inner balance of the West, with which intellectual knowledge denies the Divine, or even considers a divine core of the world impossible

"Faith" is not an intellectual "holding true" but a living inner certainty of a Great One.

Friedrich von Schiller, doctor, poet, philosopher and historian, sees cultivation of emotional sensibility in comparison to the above- mentioned Enlightenment movement as the more urgent need of the time

He translated the sapere aude[73] as "be bold with wisdom".

Schiller noted that all enlightenment of the mind deserves respect only insofar as it flows back to the character. It also starts from the character, because the way to the head has to be opened through the heart. Formation of the faculty of sensation, then, is the more urgent need of the time, not only because it becomes a means to make the improved insight for life effective, but because it awakens to the improvement of insight.

The improvement of insight leads – as mentioned above and explained by Krishna in the Bhagavadgita – to wisdom, which includes immediate comprehension and intuition. Here I come back to the person who rests in the Self (Swasthya) and lives in the consciousness (Buddhi).

In order to avoid misunderstandings, terms such as Chitta (unconsciousness, also attachment to the higher consciousness), Manas (mind) and Ahamkara (self-consciousness in the sense of ego) are explained in this context. [74]

Mental functions in Ayurveda

This appears best suited by a brief description of the following mental functions:

Sattvic mental funtions
Sattvic mental functions of inner peace, joy, non-attachment, clear memory correspond to Chitta.

Sattvic mental functions of clear perception, discernment, honesty, tolerance, solid ethical rules are buddhi.

Sattvic mental functions control of the senses correspond to manas.

Sattvic mental functions spiritual concept of self-giving, respect for all living beings correspond to Ahamkara.

Rajasic mental functions

Rajasic mental functions of worry, desire, irritability, anger are in line with Chitta.

Rajasic mental functions critical mind, opinionated, judgmental, narrow-minded correspond to Buddhi.

Rajasic mental functions many desires, aggression, competitiveness, willpower correspond to manas.

Rajasic mental functions ambitious, overbearing, vain, complacent correspond to Ahamkara.

Tamasic mental functions

Tamasic mental functions deep-seated blockages and arrests, depression, hate feelings correspond to Chitta.

Tamasic mental functions of deep-seated prejudice, dishonesty, adherence to one's own opinion, disappointment are buddhi.

Tamasic mental functions easily influenced, endless pondering, entangled in violent sensations, drug addiction correspond to Manas.

Tamasic mental factors negative image of oneself, fears, dependence correspond to Ahamkara.

Buddhi corresponds analogously with Noesis, by which Plato understands the highest cognitive faculty, which captures unchangeable truth directly and realistically, independently of any sensory perception.

To overcome the destructive ego and return to Buddhi, the transpersonal mental faculty of the mind, can be compared here to the restoration of humanity in the sense of Fritjof Capra.

How the characteristics can be positively used and developed is explained in more detail in the concluding chapter.

At this point the term swasthya should be further examined.

Resting in swasthya, an expression of health in Ayurveda, presuppose self-development.

What can be understood by this?

In this context the term individuation mentioned earlier in this book is explained in more detail here. The Latin origin of individuare means to make indivisible, to become inseparable.

What is meant is a process of becoming whole, of something unique, of an individual. The process of "becoming one's self" is the unfolding of one's own potential within one's own possibilities through the gradual awareness and realization of one's uniqueness.

C. G. Jung puts it this way: "Individuation means becoming a single being and, insofar as we understand by individuality our innermost, ultimate and incomparable uniqueness, to become our own self. One could therefore translate ‚individuation' as ‚self-fulfillment' or as ‚self-realization'. [75]

The outcome and the goal of the lifelong individuation process is the self. Gradually, more and more areas of unconsciousness are being integrated into consciousness created through new and more comprehensive adaptation.

Jung distinguishes the innate possibility of individuation from the consciously grasped and lived spiritual wholeness.

To illustrate, M. L. von Franz, a research associate of Carl Gustav Jung, refers to the image of a mountain pine with all its possibilities already in the seed. [76]

The holistic nature of this pine responds to special circumstances such as the nature of the earth, inclination of the slope, wind conditions, etc., and develops into a unique, unrepeatable, single pine, which is the only real one, for the pine itself is only the tree's possibility.

If the person becomes aware of this growth, he experiences this growth process as a reality in which he can participate, according to Jung, through free decision of the will.

This event, described by Jung as an individuation process in the real sense, is in the human being more than the whole nucleus and circumstances of fate working together.

An invisible creative influence intervenes here in a personally individual way. However, one can only come closer to the actual deeper meaning by liberating each useful thought, every purposeful thought.

This aspect of liberation, of letting go is also emphasized in several places in the Bhagavad Gita.

For example, in the 6th and 18th chapters [77]: "Srībhagavānuvāca anāśritaḥ karmaphalaṃ kāryaṃ karma karoti yaḥsa saṃnyāsī"

Krishna said: Whoever fulfills the duty imposed on him, without clinging to the fruits of his actions, is a sannyasin (one who has released, one who is free).

Even a sattvic actor is perfect in the sense that he is free from egoism and attachment, unaffected by success or failure, bestowed with enthusiasm and determination.

The process of self-realization involves both the conscious and, to a greater extent, the unconscious.

According to C. G. Jung "when the consciousness participates actively and experiences and at least understands each step of the process, then the next image begins in each case on the higher level gained thereby, and thus the direction of the goal arises." [78]

4. Prevention and self-healing – Cornerstones of Ayurveda

At the beginning of this chapter, it should be emphasized once again that the following contribution in this book should not be construed as a guide or recommendation for self-healing and is not a replacement for a visit to the doctor in the presence of any of the diseases shown here.

The explanations are merely informative ayurvedic assessment and appropriate treatment of the neurological disorders described here by way of example.

The following remarks may provide an insight into how complex ayurvedic therapies interact with each other and how they interact in a synergistic way.

Ayurveda as a holistic medicine argues that the human being in its entirety must be regarded as a unity of body, soul and spirit in its relation to the natural, social, man-made and supersensible environment in its entirety and not just in its sub-aspects.

"The whole is more than the sum of its parts". [79]

For the reader of the Western Hemisphere, some of the ayurvedic therapies presented here may seem strange and even disgusting, such as "gomutra," whereby apart from other medicines cow`s urine is administered for treatment of depression.

Other ayurvedic treatments, such as nasal rinsing (nasyam) and various enemas (basti) may also appear to the Western reader as a quackery lacking in scientific studies and thus scientifically proven efficacy.

At this point, I kindly ask the interested reader, unaffected by prejudices, fixed patterns of thinking and conditioned behaviors, to become more familiar with the deeper background of the ayurvedic applications just mentioned.

Ayurveda is an empirical science that has implemented curative measures over several millennia of insights in an open medical system.

Preventive measures are the first and most urgent concern of Ayurveda. In the case of a disease holistic measures are considered, taking into account body, mind and soul of the affected person individually according to constitution and according to his social environment.

Chronic diseases have not set in "overnight" but have evolved over time due to certain negative exogenous and endogenous factors. The cause of the disease is rarely proven to be mono-causal, but rather hides in multi-causal facets that engage interactively as the modern medical direction of psycho-neuro-endocrine immunology has recognized (as mentioned above).

Ayurveda does not treat symptoms of a disease, but applies a range of measures that address the cause.

Using the examples of manic depression (bipolar affective disorder) and strong depressive episode, I try to explain the rationality of the various Ayurvedic applications.

Health is contentment, illness is discontent

Before that, a few clarifying thoughts on health and illness seem appropriate, which I begin with the following succinct definition of Caraka: "Health is contentment, illness is discontent." [80]

This shrewd definition, given about two thousand five hundred years ago by Caraka, one of the great Indian physicians and author of the Samhita, the fundamental work of internal medicine, may at first seem superficial.

On closer inspection, however, this Vedic knowledge, which is condensed to the essential, proves to be concentrated knowledge, which requires an explanation.

Synonymous with contentment are understood among others the following terms: frugality, cheerfulness, life affirmation, serenity, modesty, confidence, harmony, cheerfulness, bliss, peace, courage, basic trust, wellbeing, joy, friendship, harmony, balance.

Could Caraka be interpreted as having health in the presence of these characteristics, and having disease in the presence of opposite characteristics?

Excursus regarding happiness, health, longevity:

Among other things, the lifestyle of the Danish people should be pointed out, since the lifestyle of this people allows revealing conclusions about the quality of life of its inhabitants and thus of the individual citizen.

According to the World Happiness Report prepared for the United Nations, the Danes are one of the happiest peoples in the world despite the dark winter months that actually favor SAD (winter depression).

The happiness report analyzes social and economic survey data of individual countries, such as income, freedom of choice, working conditions and health. [81]

In addition to these factors, other areas such as social justice, perceived corruption in the public sector, labor market access and future prospects for children and adolescents play an important role in the happiness of a people.

According to the Social Justice Index 2017, Denmark ranks first with 7.39 points in the twenty-eight EU countries, with an EU average of 5.85.

Denmark also ranks first in the index "Access to the labor market and future prospects for children and young people".[82]

In the Corruption Perception Index/CPI – perceived corruption in the public sector – of one hundred and seventy-four examined countries in 2014 among civil servants and politicians, Denmark achieves a high integrity value with ninety-two of one hundred achievable index points, thus being largely free from corruption. A value of zero index points expresses a very corrupt perception. [83]

These examples already give an indication why a people like the Danes can be described as happy. This can be clearly explained by the core element of the Danish tradition, which is expressed in the phenomenon "hygge".

The Danes consider themselves social beings whose contentment is expressed in close relationships. The most important social and close relationships are those that you experience together with others. Understanding the experience of sharing thoughts and feelings and giving and receiving support is in one word: "hygge".[84]

Hygge is a typical lifestyle of the Danes, characterized by a warm atmosphere that shares the good in life with nice people. Friends, neighbors and last but not least the family belong to hygge, with whom one likes to eat and drink together extensively, leaving plenty of time for a stimulating conversation, leaving out the irritant issues such as politics and religion.

However, the question arises, are the happiest people also the healthiest and the ones who live longest?

The assumption suggests that the happy Danes have the longest life expectancy in the world. However, this is not the case. The Danes rank 27th and live on average just over a year longer than the Americans. [85]

The Danes smoke a lot and consume a lot of meat and sugar, which is not compatible with a long and healthy life.

So it is not surprising that the Danes in the health sector reach only ninth place within the twenty-eight EU countries.

Denmark is even worse off in some areas of the health sector, such as cancer and respiratory disease as causes of death.

After Hungary, according to a statistic of the standardized mortality rate of the EU countries, Denmark has the second highest rate for cancer as the cause of death and the third highest rate for respiratory diseases. [86]

Can a people really be happy despite this unfortunate health situation? According to Caraka, this seems contradictory. So the question is whether the definition of happiness underlying the UN report is apt to really show the deeper meaning of happiness?

Happiness, as measured in the World Happiness Report – in terms of income, freedom of choice, working conditions, carefree life in material wealth – may be too one-sidedly oriented toward the values of the civilized world, disregarding important measures of values of indigenous peoples, who may have a very different and deeper understanding of happiness.

The following example of the way of life and lifestyle of a small people (or tribe) on the Macai River in the Amazon region of Brazil certainly cannot be adopted by the rest of the world, but may raise some interesting questions and provide answers, such as how the civilized world's lifestyle can adopt positive aspects of the Pirahã who live there, which have become lost to the civilized world. They live on a tributary of the Amazon two day trips by boat from the outer edges of civilization, still today largely without civilizational achievements, without electricity, without telephone and without a doctor.

The linguistics professor Daniel Everett lived for three decades with the Pirahã and was enthusiastic about their unusual perception of the world, in which there are no numbers, no descriptions of the past, hardly any concepts for the abstract. The Pirahã also engage in regular dialogue with ghosts.

Everett, in his book "The Happiest People" [87], describes how the Pirahãs lead a life in the here and now, which also shapes their language according to the principle of immediate experience. Towards death, these people show a stoic attitude. Ideas for an abstract authority are more amusing. Everett is particularly impressed by the cheerfulness of these Indians. Even in mishaps there is happiness and good humor. They are full of confidence; worries about the future are as good as unknown.

Everett concludes, "And the quality of their soul life, their happiness, and their contentment speak for their values."

What can the modern industrial and service society adopt from this to improve their quality of life? To be converted by an Indian tribe far from civilization, is that possible? Can modern people find their way back to this primitive trust that protects them, not afraid of death, even in the case of mishaps, keeping happiness and a good mood, full of confidence and without worrying about the future?

Here aspects are addressed that were at best only touched upon by the standards of value in the World Happiness Report but are indispensable for happiness in the deeper sense.

Two points from the Bhagavad Gita and the Caraka Samhita outline the deeper meaning of these aspects.

Thus the enlightened one is called someone whose mind is not disturbed by grief and distress, who does not fall into despondency when misfortune befalls him[88] You do not achieve big goals in any future coming soon. Sorrowful thinking tends to distract from the only real goal of uniting with the true inner self. [89]

The wise man is not subject to the delusion that he is a material body. This delusion is the actual epitome of the ego. [90]

Caraka [91] sees misery grounded in a false idea of "being-mine". When, in the following, the knowledge grows, when one knows that one is not the body, when one overcomes the >mine< the knower transcends everything with this truth.

This is very similar to the life attitude of the Pirahã, who lead a life in the here and now, showing a stoic attitude towards death, maintaining a good mood in times of mishaps, and almost unfamiliar with worries about the future.

Compare also the Bible passage Matthew 6, 25/26 "Therefore I say to you: Do not worry about your life, what you will eat and drink, not even on your body, what you will wear. Is not life more than food and the body more than the clothes? Look at the birds under the sky: they do not sow, they do not reap, they do not gather in the barns; and your Heavenly Father nourishes them. Are not you much more than they? "

From these life-conceptions shown by examples, a universal principle may possibly be discerned in the deeper core, which opens the door to the perfection of the human being.

To what extent this attitude is expressed in Ayurveda and Yoga is of universal importance, I will try to represent in the final chapter.

Here I stretch a bow and quote Caraka again: "Health is contentment, illness is discontent."

The importance and the realization that satisfied people generally show no pathological symptoms, is remarkably also used as a criterion in modern psychotherapy. [92]

It should be mentioned here that Ayurveda or Yoga differs significantly from modern psychoanalysis, since the study of negative psychological patterns and the psychological analysis of their formation alone do not solve these problems.

Frawley points out that, on the other hand, a mantra can change the vibrational pattern of consciousness and thus negate negative psychic patterns. [93]

A mantra changes the energetic structure in the mental field in a positive way and is therefore suitable for solving the problem.

So much for Caraka and the concise juxtaposition of contentment and health.

The classical Ayurvedic definition of health describes various requirements of health. These were formulated by Sushruta, the Indian surgeon and presumptive author of Sushruta Samhita Sutrasthana, which together with the Caraka Samhita is one of the first texts of Ayurvedic medicine [94]:

"Sama dosha sama agnisha sama dhatu mala kriyaaha prasanna atma indriya manaha swasthya iti abhidheeyate."

In detail, therefore, the conditions for health are these: Balance of the doshas. With dosha, the functional principles in the body (Vata, Pitta and Kapha) are addressed, which determine all the physiological, psychological and spiritual aspects of one's own life.

Ayurveda describes in detail how they are subtly intertwined with their five subdivisions and can be kept in balance, in normal state of tissues (dhatus) and excretions (malas) and metabolic processes (agni).

Ayurveda regards healthy excretory functions as an essential prerequisite for perfect health. In addition to the intake and digestion of food and fluid, the intestine plays a crucial role in the defense against harmful substances and pathogens. The various tasks are then accomplished in the best possible way when the intestinal mucosa, the intestine-associated immune system and the intestinal flora are optimally coordinated.

Prerequisites for health are above all normal sensory functions (indriya), intact body intelligence, well-being of the mind (manaha) and a happy soul (atma).

When, finally, inner contentment, harmony of soul, spirit and senses, as well as social well-being determine life in an all-encompassing way, the person rests in its pivot, in swasthya and enjoys optimal health.

It should be mentioned that more than seventy years ago, the World Health Organization (WHO) expressed a positive and holistic understanding of health in its definition of health. This definition goes far beyond the biomedical approach, which describes health as a condition in which diseases and pathological changes cannot be detected. [95]

WHO: "Health is a state of complete physical, mental and social well-being and not just the absence of disease or affliction." [96]

The scientifically understood narrow concept of health according to the bio-medical model "as the absence of disease" is today confronted with a holistic concept of health. Health can refer to the individual, and be understood as a state of physical and mental well-being, or of physical and mental functioning and efficiency.

According to the understanding of the social and health scientist Klaus Hurrelmann, health is a pleasant and not at all natural state of equilibrium of risk and protection factors, which is questioned again and again at every biographical point in time.

If the balance is achieved, meaning and joy can be gained from life, a productive development of one's own competences and performance potentials is possible, and the willingness increases to integrate and engage socially. [97]

The definition of health formulated by Hurrelmann is generally understood to be a consistent evolution of the WHO definition mentioned above and is now used by all disciplines of health sciences.

This concept is also close to the view of Antonovsky, who uses the expression "sense of coherence" in the context of salutogenesis (development of health). By recognizing and understanding protection and risk factors the individual's own life seems to be meaningful and capable of being influenced.

A person with a pronounced sense of coherence possesses a positive self-image and self-confidence and is able to gain joy and meaning from life and promotes the creative realization of one's own performance potential.

At the same time, the willingness for social integration and commitment increases and also, according to the psychologist and happiness researcher Mihaly Cscikzentmihalyi, human well-being. [98]

"Our well-being increases when we use our energy for goals that go beyond the moment and self-interest.

Tracking short-term goals makes us happier than not pursuing any goals; pursuing long-term goals makes us happier than pursuing short-term goals; working on one's own perfection makes us happier than any amusements, and one's commitment to the well-being of another person or group makes us happier than the commitment to egocentric goals."

As explained later, contentment, well-being, and their just-mentioned associated concepts are the purposes of yogic practice in the endeavor to ultimately achieve spiritual perfection.

Just as health represents a pleasant and by no means self-evident state of equilibrium, which is always questioned at every point in the history of life, the happiness experience also behaves.

If one succeeds in keeping the balance, then meaning and joy can be gained from life

Happiness and contentment, as well as health, is not the natural state that suits you, but something that you have to work hard to achieve. To be happy and to feel contented are inner states - and they are easily transient.

Everyone is not through luck born a blacksmith, but everyone can become through luck a blacksmith.

To understand luck, here's an entertaining anecdote by Gary Player, a world-class golfer, quoted in an interview published in Golf Digest Magazine in 2002. [99]

"I practiced in a sand bunker in Texas and this good old boy with a big hat stopped to watch me. The first shot he saw went into the hole.

He said, "You get 50 bucks if you knock the next one in." I also holed the next one.

Then he said, "You will get $ 100 if you also hole the next one."

That went as well; there were three in a row.
    As he settled the bill, he said, "Boy, I've never seen anyone so lucky in my life." And I shot back: "Well, the harder I practice, the luckier I get."

Swasthya – Rest in Self

Satisfaction and happiness do not come automatically; it is the basic attitude to life, to control inner experiences and to be able to process negative experiences in a positive way.
    This basic attitude is expressed in Ayurveda by Swasthya (resting in self). Swasthya is also the ayurvedic key word for health.
    In order to understand more deeply the meaning of swasthya, one should deal with what is meant by self. Who are you, what are you and why are you are questions whose answers can bring you closer to realization.
    Svasthya derives from the Sanskrit term Sva, meaning to belong to oneself. In this context, swasthya means self-assurance, self-esteem, self-confidence and, most importantly, basic trust.

The latter includes both trust in oneself (I feel sheltered), trust in others (I trust the partnership) and trust in the world (life is worth living).

Basic trust thus enables a fearless confrontation with the social environment.

There are numerous descriptions for swasthya, such as well-being, contentment (Santosha in Yoga), prosperity, determination, state of self-realization, state of self-restraint.

In the final chapter "Ayurveda and Yoga - the magic connection", the term Santosha - the joy that springs from an inner serenity - is explained in more detail in the context of Patanjali's Yogasutras.

To recognize and to live according to one's own nature is the prerequisite and goal for a fulfilled life. As long as we stay in touch with our true self - our innermost nature - our personality rests in serenity and cannot be shaken by anything.

The moment a person remembers an experience in the past or becomes aware of a project in the future, the experience of his living pure being becomes the imagination of his person as the center of an event.

If, on the other hand, when he remembers a flash of the self that he experienced, then that memory becomes present again at the same moment. For the self as absolute consciousness is timeless and spaceless. A parallel statement can be found in the Bible "Only the eternal will remain, which cannot be shaken".[100]

That's what I think comes closest to the Self. This imperturbability of a tiny living being in an immeasurable universe, touched by an idea of the Eternal Being and, through a feeling of life beyond the senses and the mind, to be deeply connected with the hidden seed of all being, to require no further possessions, totally free, to be filled with bliss.

Worth mentioning are still today's terms, such as "flow effect" and "Oneness", which correspond to supreme moments of happiness.

According to the already mentioned Csiskszentmihàlyi, who is also acknowledged to be an outstanding scientist in the field of flow theory, flow effect is reached by the highest form of concentration and self-forgetfulness, whereby subjectively a fusion with the environment is felt. After reaching that goal enhancement and self-expansion is relived. [101]

For "Oneness" Roger Gabriel (Raghavanand) sets for me a very vivid consideration. [102]

"What is Oneness?

Imagine that you are the whole universe. You live in complete joy and bliss. Imagine, there is no past or future, only now. Imagine, there is no space or time, just an infinite eternity. Imagine endless peace, harmony and unconditional love. Imagine no fear, imagine equality in all things. That is oneness.

Unfortunately we can never imagine that fully. To understand or experience something, we have to compare it to something else, which immediately brings us into duality. Unity is incomparable by definition.

So is it possible to know Oneness?

Yes, but only through direct experience, when we go beyond the mind, the intellect and the ego. Unity is the coming together of all opposites.

It is always with us as the basis and underlying essence of everything. It's nothing in itself, but contains the potential for everything.

We have to go beyond the senses, beyond duality, to find oneness."

The following inspirational Vedanta quote may conclude those thoughts:

"The ignorant (absorbed in duality) wants material wealth, the intelligent (seeker on the way) wants enlightenment, but the sage (the connoisseur of Oneness) loves and receives everything."

So much for prevention and health, let's turn to the ayurvedic concept of disease.

Note:
The following statements may be of particular interest to one or the other reader. For the unprejudiced reader, the remarks may seem quite abstract and therefore only "flown over".

However, they serve the purpose of clarifying the complex course of ayurvedic diagnosis and therapy, and so I hope that these representations are also observed by the readers mentioned last.

The remarks on manic-depressive illness and on severe depressive episode, which are presented in later sections, intend to provide an overview of the extremely versatile treatment of ayurvedic medicine in such diseases.

Recognizing causes of illness

How does Ayurveda react to a case of illness?

In case of illness Ayurveda tries to recognize the spiritual and emotional background of the illness. A significant part of the illness is due to mental causes. Causes are mostly wrong thought patterns, unprocessed emotional impressions and negative expressions of the psyche.

Ayurveda helps in the holistic sense to become aware of the coarse and subtle connections between man and nature and thus leads to healing. In addition ayurvedic healing applications open the view to the spiritual dimension, beyond space and time.

Ayurveda has a deep understanding of the disease and its timing and history, which is reflected in six disease phases (see below).

Preceded is a verse from classical Ayurveda [103]:

"Janmaantara kritam paapam vyaadhi roopena bhaadate, Tat shantihi aushadhaihi, daanaihi, japa homa suaarchanaihi."

All diseases are rooted in the mind before they manifest. The mind has a longer shelf life than the physical body. The imprints of the mind are transferred to the next body.

In this context, the subject of reincarnation, Karma and vedic astrology is of importance, which cannot be dealt with in the context of this book.

It should be mentioned, however, that the Bhagavadgita emphasizes the mental and emotional connection between health and illness. Those who follow and encourage negative forces (Adharma) develop suffering, and those who follow positive forces (Dharma) keep the entire life-flow in harmony. [104]

Diseases are defined in Ayurveda as a disharmony of internal balance. They always start when our natural state of health (prakriti) comes into contact with a disease-causing factor, which disturbs our balance.

The constitution is inflicted (vikriti) and the person suffers from the resulting illness of a physical and psychological nature.

Diseases manifest themselves in imbalances of the sensitive external aura (energetic envelope) long before physical symptoms are discernible. For example, this manifests itself among other things in diminishing joie de vivre. We sense that something is wrong.

Physicians cannot detect any "organic" abnormalities with their means. Psychologists try to approach the problem with intellectually oriented means.

It is remarkable that Ayurveda can detect early on emerging diseases in the first stages. Ayurveda tries to correct the recognizable imbalance in time to bring the body back into balance.

Herein lies the important preventative approach of Ayurvedic medicine.

If there is no change in the way of life, the disturbances spread to denser emotional energy fields. The symptoms increase and eventually manifest in the physical area. First, individual cells are affected, then organs, and finally the whole body.

Diseases are usually due to the complex networked control circuits of the organism, not triggered off by a single cause.

Disease-causing factors

General causes:
- excessive, too little or other abusive use of the senses (exaggerated, apathy, drug abuse)
- wrong physical and / or mental diet (junk food / black magic)
- unhealthy working conditions and stressful social environment. (Dust, gases, noise, bad air)
- chaotic lifestyle (irregular daily routine, disorder, over-stimulation, insomnia)
- excessive stress (burnout)
- extremely pronounced seasons (extreme heat, cold, humidity or extreme drought)

Suffering of the spirit (five sufferings - Panchaklesha):

- Ignorance   Avidya
- Selfishness   Asmita
- Attachment   Raga
- Dislike   Devesha
- Fear of death   Ahhinivesha

All these factors, to a certain extent, represent an excessive demand for the organism, which inevitably leads to a disturbance of the structural and functional components in the body.

Various signs (Purvaroopa) are to be recognized as warnings and whistle-blowers at an early stage and treated before the disease can accumulate in the body.

For example, diffuse symptoms such as flatulence and constipation, which cannot yet be attributed to any defined disease, are to be taken as omens.

If the disease has already established itself in the body, main symptoms (Roopa) are shown, which indicate the extent of the doshas involved in the disease's development. Depending on the phase of the disease, specific treatability is determined.

Disease phases (Kriyakala)

Ayurveda distinguishes the following six disease phases:
1. Accumulation   Sanchaya
2. Provocation   Prakopa
3. Spread   Prasara
4. Localization   Sthana Samshraya
5. Manifestation   Vyakti
6. Chronic Presence   Bheda

Kriyakala, a combination of words from Kriya (action) and Kala (time) can be understood as "the time to act".

By the time of the Prakopa stage, health can be fully restored by taking appropriate measures.

Occasionally, spontaneous remissions (Prashama) also occur when the doshas regain their equilibrium for seasonal reasons. For example, if after a "winter depression" (SAD) disorders of the biological circadian rhythm are lifted by days with longer incidence of light.

If the omens are ignored, the imbalance of the doshas will increase and thus the untreated disease process will reach the next disease stages.

1) Accumulation (Samchaya)
By accumulation Ayurveda in this context means the accumulation of a dosha at its specific seat in the body. For example, with Vata in the large intestine (constipation), Pitta in the stomach (heartburn) and Kapha in the lungs (mucilage).

In this case, the multiplication is faster or stronger than the body can eliminate the accumulation. The respective main seats of the Doshas are of Vata the large intestine, the bladder and kidneys, of Pitta the lower stomach, small intestine, liver, pancreas and of Kapha the chest, head, neck and upper stomach.

The first signs at this stage may be nonspecific symptoms, such as malaise or mild discomfort in the appropriate body region.

In the initial stages, the disorders can be corrected and remedied with simple measures, since the Dhatus (body tissues), Malas (excreta) and Srotas (body channels) have not yet been damaged. If the diseases have manifested in the body, further therapeutic measures are necessary.

As a rule, in the case of a short-term disturbance, the body recovers its balance thanks to its self-healing power.

For example, after a rich high fat and carbohydrate meal, digestive disorders usually occur, such as bloating, discomfort, flatulence.

Reacting to this with balanced food intake and physical activity, the natural balance is restored. Maintaining the luscious diet can lead to further symptoms and usually long-term illnesses.

2) Provocation (Prakopa)
If the apparent imbalance has not been counteracted, deterioration will now follow. The symptoms are more noticeable but are often ignored at this stage. Thus, a person suffering from an upset stomach gets an acute irritation of the stomach by maintaining a poor diet.

3) Scattering / propagation (Prasara)
At this stage dosha accumulation begins to spread from the local source and spreads to other parts of the body with associated complications in other parts of the body.

At this stage, changes in lifestyle, such as improved nutrition, are generally no longer sufficient but require additional therapies. For example, selected herbal preparations are administered.

4) Localization / Fixing (Sthana-Samsraya)
In this early stage of a disease, the migratory doshas settle in a particular tissue or organ.

While the prevalence of the dominant doshas has not been alleviated so far, migratory doshas usually settle to develop additional symptoms in certain tissues and other organ systems at this early stage of the disease.

As a result, the association with causative dosha accumulation may be overlooked, and the new symptoms may be addressed as a separate imbalance.

A disorder of the doshas is expressed by various symptoms:

Excessive Vata is manifested by emaciation, weakness, trembling, nervousness, anxiety, distention of the bladder and constipation, sleep disturbances, disorientation, dizziness, confusion, depression.

Excess pitta is expressed by the yellow color of the eyes, the skin, the urine, excrement, also by hunger, thirst, heartburn and sleep problems.

Excess Kapha can be detected by lower digestive power, nausea, lethargy, lack of exercise, heaviness, white color, cough, difficulty in breathing, chills and excessive sleep.[105]

5) Manifestation (Vyakti)

At this stage, specific symptoms of a manifested disease are prominent, such as edema (sopha), fever (jvara) or diarrhea (atisara).

Beginning with this stage, the symptoms are so pronounced that they are generally no longer neglected, but a doctor is consulted.

6) Chronic presence (Bheda)

In the Bheda stage it emerges whether a disease becomes chronic or incurable.

In this last phase of the ayurvedic stages of the disease, the imbalance of the doshas has spread so far that it can lead to a chronification of the symptoms and complications. Structural changes to the organs may have already occurred and provoked another disease.

Frequently, diseases are detected only at this late stage. This is the case, for example, for the metabolic disease type 2 diabetes mellitus, when much damage has already occurred in the body.

Effects of deterioration

Increased Vata leads to detachment of the mind from the body and disorientation. There is a nervous over-activity at the expense of a balanced flow of juices, the body begins to degenerate.

Increased Pitta leads to an accumulation of internal heat and fever with inflammation and infections.

Increased Kapha leads to weight gain and heaviness in the body, apathy and lethargy.

So much for recognizing general causes of illness. The descriptions may have provided certain basic knowledge that may facilitate the understanding of the following remarks for the evaluation of some major diseases and disorders of psychic and neurological genesis from the Ayurvedic point of view.

Psychiatric syndromes

The following depiction and description of some of the psychiatric symptoms enumerated by Caraka may serve as an introduction to the complexity of the sufferings of mental and neurological origins. By discussing some of these psychiatric symptoms, it is intended to highlight various negative factors that can lead to severe neurotic disorders, such as manic depressive disorder (bipolar affective disorder) or severe depressive episodes.

In the following section, etiological factors, pathology and the various extensive therapeutic measures for the treatment of manic-depressive disorder and severe depressive episode are presented from the ayurvedic perspective.

Through many years of contact with my naturopath colleagues in the German Naturopathic Association (Bundesverband freier Heilpraktiker e.V.), I have been inspired by interest in a presentation of appropriate ayurvedic therapies. I kindly ask the uninhibited reader to understand that I am dealing with this issue here, especially since I assume that some of the explanations are also of general interest.

First of all, Ayurveda distinguishes between diseases of primary mental origin and predominantly mental symptoms (Kevala Manasika Rogas) and diseases of primary mental origin and predominantly of physical symptoms (Mano-Sharirika / psychosomatic disorders). [106]

For example, the first mentioned group, which is influenced by Rajas and Tamas, includes the following emotional disturbances, some of them already mentioned by Caraka:

1. Kāma   (Lust)
2. Krodha   (Anger)
3. Lobha   (Greed)
4. Moha   (Delusion)
5. Irshya   (Jealousy)
6. Mana   (Pride)
7. Chittodvega   (Mania, Fear)
8. Chinta   (Depression)

To the psychosomatic disorders under the influence of Rajas, Tamas and Vata, Pitta and Kapha Ayurveda assigns the following afflictions:

1. Unmāda / Insanity. Ayurveda assigns three meanings to the state of insanity, such as: Buddhivikara (deformity of the will), Manovikara (deformity of the mind) and Atmavikara (deformity of the intellect) [107]
2. Apasmāra (epilepsy)
3. Apatantraka (apoplectic fits / stroke)
4. Bhayaja and Śokaja Atisāra (diarrhea due to fear and sadness)
5. Kāmaja and Śokajajwara (nervous pyrexia)
6. Nidranāśa
7. Shandha

A person afflicted by these mental disorders or diseases is practically a prisoner who has lost his knowledge of his true self and whose life is largely determined by the afflictions just mentioned.

If, on the other hand, the affected person deals with these internal enemies and becomes aware of the destructive driving forces, this is the first step towards improvement and the path to self-knowledge and self-healing.

To (1) Kāma (Lust)

According to Hinduism, Kāma (worldly desire) is one of the four life goals (Purusharthas) of man and desirable as long as Kāma is subordinate to other life goals, such as Dharma (a life according to cosmic laws), Moksha (salvation) and Artha (prosperity and success).

If worldly pleasure is out of control, for example through insatiable desire, it shows itself to be an evil of a lower human nature.

Man is driven by his ego to fulfill his own needs through constant pursuit of self-satisfaction. He is dominated by the lowest instincts that cause suffering. [108] This type of ailment constitutes a psychiatric syndrome.

To (2) Krodha (Anger):

Kāma evolves from the Raja Guna (Passion) and is constantly driven to satisfy the insatiable desires. Since this does not succeed Kāma takes the form of Krodha (anger). [109]

According to the Hindu scriptures, Kāma and Krodha are two major passions of the six inner enemies (Arishadvargas), which include Lobha (greed), Moha (delusion), Moda (pride) and Matsarya (envy). [110]

Neither Kāma nor Krodha can be satisfied or appeased since Kama has an insatiable appetite and can never be satisfied and Krodha represents a terrible and unpredictable temperament.

If, on the basis of this knowledge, man strives with a strong will to overcome these vices through bhakti (loving care) and abstention, he can free himself from the grip of these constraints. On the path of self-realization, he develops the sattva Guna (goodness) and proportionally reduces Kama and Krodha. After all, man identifies with his true SELF and becomes part of his own destiny.

To (3) Lobha (Greed)

Lobha means greed and avarice, also impatience and confusion. Here, too, it is important to realize why one is ruled by Lobha to the point of frustration. The driving force is the unfulfilling gratification of one's own interests that cannot be satisfied. When a goal is attained, an incessant urge up to an obsession demands to possess and enjoy more.

As with Kama, the behavior is determined by Raja Guna. The preponderance of passion requires more and more, even if it is not needed anymore. Not only material abundance, but also admiration, social status and other immaterial motives can be the uncontrollable driving forces.

The subsequent well-known saying attributed, among others, to the American comedian Danny Kaye, illustrates the absurdity of Lobha:

"Time and again, man spends money he does not have, for things he does not need, to impress people who he does not like."

Lobha, especially the personally motivated, selfish greed, has to be overcome. As mentioned above, according to Csikszentmihalyi, our well-being increases as we use our energy for purposes beyond the moment and self-interest. An antidote to breaking away from Lobha is the yogic practice of Santosha (contentment), as explained in more detail in the last chapter.

To (4) Moha (Delusions)

Moha refers to what conflicts with knowledge. The person bound to his lust and longings lives in an illusion in this material world. Tempted by delusions, he sees enemies everywhere in the outer world.

True knowledge, on the other hand, comes about through gaining control over the internal enemies.

Incidentally, above the archway of the Holstentor, the landmark of the Free and Hanseatic City of Lübeck, the inscription "Concordia domi foris pax" in golden letters welcomes entrants in an appropriate way meaning "Concord at home – peace outside".

Again, it is expressed that the internal enemies such as sensual desire, lust, anger, greed, envy and misconception are the cause of the emergence of external enemies.

In other words, by controlling the internal enemies, the submission of the external enemies is achieved. [111]

To (5) Irshya (Jealousy)

The Sanskrit term for jealousy is Irshya, Matsarya or Asuya. However, there is a subtle difference. While Matsarya means stinginess and the basis for not being able to let go of the material things of life, jealousy is a special kind of emotion or vritti that arises in the Rajasic mind, where the person concerned looks on enviously at wealth, success or higher virtuous qualities of others. Manifestations of jealousy are hatred and envy. One person, filled with these negative qualities, tries to hurt a supposedly better person by gossip, slander and other accusations. [112]

The mind becomes what it thinks about.

Therefore one should think about thinking, as the following aphorism teaches.[113]

Watch your thoughts,

because they become feelings.

Watch your feelings,

because they become words.

Watch your words,

because they become actions.

Watch your actions,

because they become habits.

Pay attention to your habits,

because they become your character.

Watch your character

because it will be your destiny.

For example, those who perceive predominantly negative things, whose brains are trimmed to this selective perception, conceal at the same time pleasant things. The focus is permanently on the negative and makes them sick in the long run. Negative thoughts – plagued by jealousy – are also the driving force of a degenerate mind.

Negative thinking of a jealousy-filled person can only be changed by cultivating the opposite. This is helped by the yogic practice of Pratipaksha Bhavana. This will be discussed in more detail in the final chapter.

The Sanskrit word Pratipaksha means opposite, and the Sanskrit word Bhavana means cultivation. To cultivate are therefore the virtuous qualities opposed to jealousy, such as nobleness or magnanimity.

When nobleness comes to the place, jealousy goes out by itself.

To (6) Mana (Pride)

Mana is a Sanskrit term with multiple meanings. Mana can mean healthy self-esteem, self-respect, but also in exaggerated form it can represent pride, self-importance even arrogance.

The exaggerated manifestation is described in the Bhagavad Gita: [114] Chapter 16, verse 17 as follows: Self-possessed, stubborn, intoxicated with pride in their possessions, they perform hypocritical acts of ordination, in name only, contrary to the traditional rules.

Such a mentality has succumbed to illusion, tempted by the accumulation of wealth, tempted to pride by false prestige.

To 7) Chittodvega (Mania / Anxiety)

Chitta refers to psyche and Udvega refers to fear. Fear is a vague sense of concern accompanied by one or several body sensations. As a kind of warning signal, fear is a normal response to threatening influences and is useful because it encourages the individual to take necessary measures to prevent the threat or minimize its consequences.

Episodic anxiety is usually classified as anxiety neurosis, accompanied by somatic symptoms such as palpitations, paresthesia, weakness, dizziness, pessimism and irritability, low self-esteem and nervousness.

The ayurvedic treatment of anxiety disorders (Cittodvega) therefore includes the following measures:

1. Vata regulating therapies, especially oil treatments such as forehead oil casting (Shirodhara), whole body oil casting (Pariseka), whole body oil massages (Abhyanga), ingestion of oily substances (Snehapana), exfoliation therapy (Virecana), different types of enema (Anuvasana, Yoga or Matravasti) and Nasal / sinus therapies (Nasya).

2. Conversational therapy with the help of the basic philosophical concepts of Samkhyayoga and Vedanta with corresponding exercises for the differentiation of "fear" and the perception of this anxiety.
3. Spiritual therapies to counter the prevailing Tamas with Sattva action: For example, rituals and meditative practices.
4. Avoiding Rajas and Tamas situations in all activities, especially in the diet.
5. Psycho-immunizing drugs (Medorasyana and Vajikarana) such as Withania somnifera (Ashwagandharishta, Ashwagandhadi Lehyam, Immutone) and Bacopa monnieri (Brahmarasayan, Saraswatharishta, Neurotone).

To (8) Chinta (Sad thoughts, Depression):

Depression, in Ayurveda called "dukha" (sadness), is a state of ongoing mental deprivation.

At this point, only a few general explanations are given. In more detail, depression is discussed with some of its various manifestations in the section "Manic Depressive Disorders" and "Severe Depressive Episode".

From a psychopathological aspect, depression is considered one of the affective disorders. We distinguish the depressive episode from recurrent depressive disorder and chronic illness.

The causes of depression can be exogenous (reactive, caused by a stressful event), neurotic (developmental or behavioral, such as fatigue depression) or endogenous (caused from within).

How can depression develop from the ayurvedic perspective?

From the ayurvedic-psychological point of view depression can arise from a dosha disorder, it can be karmic, triggered by certain events, arising out of neurotic involvement or arising out of exhaustion.

According to Ayurveda, depression usually develops from Vata disorders. Nevertheless, the depression may also have Pitta or Kapha character and therefore require appropriate treatment.

Assessment of some major diseases and ailments of the mind from the ayurvedic point of view

Using the example of manic-depressive illness (bipolar affective disorder) and the strong depressive episode, an assessment of these mental illnesses is given from an ayurvedic perspective.

The synergetic ayurvedic therapy methods presented here may give an impression how Ayurveda considers the interacting interweaving of body, mind and soul of man in its entirety as a living being supporting the naturally given self-healing powers.

The basis of these statements is part of a script that was kindly made available by Dr. L Mahadevan, B.A. M.S., M.D.[115]

Before that, some terms are mentioned:

As with other illnesses, the diagnosis of depression includes a detailed knowledge of the patient's medical and biographical history, current life status, and current physical and mental condition.

The World Health Organization's International Classification of Disorders (ICD-10) diagnostic system differentiates according to the number, severity and duration of certain key symptoms:

- Depressed episode in unipolar depression that may be mild, moderate or severe.
- Depressive episode in bipolar affective disorder, a condition in which depressive and manic phases alternate.
- Dysthymia, usually beginning in early adulthood, a more persistent "chronic" form of depression.

Ayurveda distinguishes the following mental dispositions - (Chitta Bhumi) and other cited features

Chitta Bhumi	Features	Predominant Guna
Kashipta (craving)	Excessive fluctuation, increased attachment to sukha and dukkha	Rajas
Mudha (forgetful)	Dull, inert Ignorance, excessive sleep	Tamas

Vikshipta (distracted)	Lack of concentration	Rajas and Tamas
Ekagara (concentrated)	Mind is purged of impurities, prolonged concentration	Satwa
Niruddha (restrained)	Calmness, tranquillity, bliss	Satwa

Personalities

Qualities of Satvic personalit	Quality of Rajasic personality	Qualities of Tamasic personality
Kindness	Unsteady nature	Despondency (dejection)
Discretion in the use of articles	Pride	Atheism
Truthfulness	Falseness	Excessive miseries
Forgiveness	Unkindness	Ignorance
Righteousness	Vanity (egoism)	Unrighteousness
Wisdom, intelligence	Pleasure	Perverted intelligence
Memory	Lust	Sleepiness
Non-attachment to worldly things	Anger	Lethargy

Types of Manobala (Mental stamina / Willpower)

Manobala	Willpower / stamina	Predominant dosha
Pravara satwa or uttama manobala	Strong willpower	Satwa
Madhyama satwa	Moderate willpower	Rajas
Avara satwa or mano dourbalyam	Weak willpower	Tamas

Etiology of Psychiatric Diseases – Ayurvedic View

Dietetic Factors	Behavioural Factors
Non Beneficial Food	Perverted Activies
Incompatible Food	Controlling natural urges
Unwholesome Food	Doing things beyond one's own capacity

Contaminated Food	Perverted Sexual activities
Untimely Food	Disrespecting elders and teachers
Toxic chemicals	
Fertilizers, non-organic food	

Types of mental diseases (Manorogam)

Unmadam	psychosis and neurosis
Apasmaram	epilepsy
Atatva abhinivesham	delusion, hallucination, illusion
Graha rogas	psychiatric and neurological disorders supposed to be caused by supernatural powers

Earlier in this book, I addressed some of the negative and positive mental factors that affect the immune system in socio-psycho-neuro-endocrine immunology. The importance of these interactions should now be considered in connection with Ayurveda.

In this section, for the evaluation and treatment of major diseases and mental diseases, examples of manic-depressive disease and strong depressive episodes are explained in detail from an ayurvedic perspective.

The focus here is on negative mental factors of the immune system. Positive mental factors influencing the immune system are in conclusion mentioned in the context of Ayurveda and Yoga.

According to ayurvedic knowledge, the following emotions lead to major diseases and mental suffering:

Kāma – lust
Krodha – anger
Lobha – greed
Moha – delusion
Matsar – jealousy

These strong emotions weaken the strength of the mind.

The Five Afflictions of the Mind (Panchaklesha)

- Ignorance- Avidya
- Egoism - Asmita
- Attachment - raga
- Aversion - Dvesha
- Strong desire to live, fear of death – Abhinivesha

A) Manic depressive disorder

Manic-depressive disease is an episodic, potentially life-long, debilitating disease that can be difficult to diagnose.

This disorder is also known as bipolar affective disorder or manic depression, characterized by episodes of raised mood (mania) usually alternating with episodes of depression.

Summary of DSM-IV-TR – Classification of Bipolar Disorder

Bipolar I	Bipolar II	Cyclothymic disorders	Bipolar Disorder Not otherwise specified
One or more manic or mixed episodes, usually accompanied by major depressive episodes MALE FEMALE	One or more manic or mixed episodes, usually accompanied by at least one hypo-manic episode FEMALE MALE	At least 2 years of numerous periods of hypo-manic and depressive symptoms *	Bipolar features that do not meet criteria for any specific bipolar disorders

*Symptoms do not meet criteria for manic and depressive episodes

Mood swings
Mania
Euthymia
Depression

Diagnostic Criteria for Manic Episodes
Three to four of the following criteria are required during the elevated mood period.

- High self-esteem
- Reduced need for sleep
- Talkativeness
- Galloping thoughts and flight of ideas
- Easily distracted, inability to maintain attention
- One-sided fixation
- Excessive commitment to pleasurable activities (sex, travel, spending money)

Etiological factors
Asatmya indriyartha Samyoga (Inappropriate contact of sensory organs)
Atiyogam (extreme use)
Ayogam (under use)
Mityayogam (abuse) of sense faculties
Prajnaparadha impairment of intellect, free will and memory
Parinama result of ill deeds leads to damage of Manas by Rajas and Tamas

Pathology - ayurvedic view
Aggravation of rajas, tamas, vata and pitta
The mind is afflicted
Mano vaha srotas (energy channels that convey thoughts, ideas, feelings and impressions) are afflicted
Chittodvegam – mania

Factors of disease development
1. *Dosa** – Manas/mind – *Raja, Tama*
2. Sarira/body – *Vata, Pitta*
3. *Dusya* – *Manas, Rasadi Sarvadhatu*
4. *Agni*/digestive capacity – *Jatharagni* – *Manda, Visama*
5. *Srotas* /channels– *Manovaha, Sarvasroto dusti*
6. *Vyakti Stana* – *Manas*
7. *Sadhyaasadhyata*/prognosis – *Kachra Sadhya* (difficult prognosis)
* A tissue (Dhatu) is in a medical view, especially in terms of treatment first and foremost a Dusya, an element of the body disfigurable by increased Dosa (Vata, Pitta, Kapha).

Therapy
- Daiva vyapasraya - Spiritual Therapy
  Mantra (incantation), mani (wearing gems),Homa (spiritual offering according to Hindu custom), etc.
- Yukti vyapasrya - Physical Therapy
  Bahya (external) and abhyantara shodhanam (internal cleansing), medhya rasayanam (brain tonic)
- Sattvavajaya - Psychotherapy
  Achara rasayanam (social and personal disciplinary programs): Explained in the final chapter (yama and niyama).

Treatment:
To reduce Vata pitta aggravation.
To reduce chala guna (restless nature) and increase of sthira guna (stability)
Madhura rasa (sweet taste) drugs
Drugs that are agni deepana – oiling to expel flatulence, (vatanulomana)
 Medhyam (brain tonics)

Formulations
  Decoctions (kashayam): 60 ml b.d. half an hour before food
- Vidryadi Kashayam (healing for rheumatic ailments)
- Dhanwantaram Kashayam (et al.)
- Bhrami drakshadi kashayam (including body burn)

Tablets (Gulika):
- Manasa mitra vatakam - 2 h.s. after food with ghee
- Dhanwantaram gulika - 2 b.d. after food

Medicated ghee (Ghrtam), dose: 10 ml h.s. with milk after food:
- Kalyanakam ghrtam
- Maha kalyanakam ghrtam
- Jeevantyadi ghrtam

Full Body Massage (Abhyangam)
- Oil = Bala laksha ashwagandhadi thailam
  (use of laksha to cure injuries, especially the nerves and ligaments is already reported in the epic Mahabharata)

- Pure sensitive oil (Shuddha bala thailam) for energy and vitality, lowers Vata and Pitta)

Fomentation (Swedanam)

Purgation (Virechanam)
Cleansing / detoxification / drainage (virechanam) with kalyanaka gulam - 30 gr, given in the morning at 9:30 on an empty stomach. It helps in cleaning of the channels (GIT in the gross level)

Yoga basti protocol: 5 basti with oil and 3 with decoction

Oil Enema	Decoction
Day	1
Day	2
Day	3
Day	4
Day	5
Day	6
Day	7
Day	8

Enema with herbal decoctions - Raja yapana

Medication/Drugs	Quantity/Amount
• honey	200 ml
• rock salt	15 gm
• Shuddha bala oil	100 ml
• Kalyanaka	100 ml
• paste from yashti madhu,	(Shatahva Peucedanaum) 30 gm
(graveolens), shyama (Setaria italica beauv), Kalinga (Holarrhena), antidys-enteruíca (preparation from Berberis arista)	
• Kshira kashayam: medicated milk,	
• Vata and Pitta soothing	300 ml
• Mamsa kahayam:	
With goat meat boiled in water	300 ml
Total amount:	**About 1000 ml**

Kaya sekam
Warm medical oil is squeezed with a rag and applied smoothly to the entire body.
Oil used:
Bala ashwagandha - lakshadi tailam.

Nasyam
Medicinal oil or herbal extracts are administered through the nose
Dose: 2 drops in each nostril
- Ksheera bala tailam
- Yashti madhu tailam

External applications
Shiro Dhara (medicated oil casting adjusted to the dosha disorder on the forehead)
with
Kshira bala oil
Bala ashwaganda oil

Shiro Basti *(head casting:*medically enriched oil adjusted to the dosha disorder is poured in an open cap)
with
Kshirabala oil
Dhanwantaram,
Bala ashwaganda lakshadi

Single medications
Ashwaganda (Withania somnifera)
Main ingredient: Withanolides
Potential medicinal properties:
- Mood stabilizer
- Rejuvenating properties (more correct: it slows down the aging process)
- Reduces oxidative stress, which can cause mental fatigue

Yashtimadhu (Glycyrrhiza glabra)
Chemical composition: Glycyrrhizc acid (GA) (main bioactive constituent of licorice)
Potential medicinal properties:

- Improve memory activity
- Cerebro protection molecule

Guduchi (Tinosporia cordifolia)
Potential medicinal properties:
- Antioxidant
- Anti-Stress
- Immunomodulatory and anti-neoplastic properties

Vidari (Pueraria tuberosa)
  Potential medicinal properties:
- Neurological protection
- Also acts as an aphrodisiac

Draksha (vitis vinifera)
  Major chemical constituents:
- Palmitic, stearic, oleic and linolenic acids, biflavonoids.
  Potential medicinal properties:
- Anti-oxidant, anti-stress activity.
- hepatoprotective,

This overview provides a first clear impression of how Ayurveda uses synergistic healing powers and activates self-healing powers.

Annotation: Manic depressive disorders - socio-political challenges
Manic-depressive disorder is one of the world's ten most common disabilities.

More research is needed to enable better detection and treatment of bipolar disorder. This is very expensive in terms of individual, economic and public health and inevitably requires the provision of adequate financial resources.

Ayurveda also strives in this area to unfold the necessary consciousness. Ayurvedic treatment provides physical, psychological and spiritual support to the patient.

Interdisciplinary cooperation of conventional medicine and Ayurveda medicine promises holistic and innovative solutions.

B) *Severe depressive episodes – Depression from the Ayurvedic point of view*

"Vishada Sarvada manah khedah". Vishada is a constant feeling of sadness and inappropriate guilt: these are the cardinal signs of depression!

DSM-IV criteria

Depressed mood and/or loss of interest
or pleasure ≥ 2 weeks duration
Associated symptoms
Physical: insomnia/hypersomnia, appetite/weight change, decreased energy, psychomotor change
Psychological: feelings of guilt or worthlessness, poor concentration/indecisiveness, thoughts
of death/suicidal intentions (SI)

A severe depressive episode is when four or more of the following symptoms are apparent:

Physical Psychological

Physical	Psychological
- Sleep disorder	- Low self-esteem
- Appetite change	- Poor concentration
- Fatigue	- Indecision
- Psychomotor retardation	- Thoughts of death

Etiological factors

Rogajam (secondary to diseases): Vishada is seen as a symptom, occasionally accompanied by hyperpyrexia due to aggravation of Vata.

In chronic conditions of mental illness and physical illness these symptoms appear combined with each other.

Samprapti / pathogenesis

Increased Kapha and Vata affect body, mind and sensory organs which eventually leads to depression (VISHADAM).

Symptoms:

1. Psychological Symptoms - Bhakti, smrti, mano Buddhi vibhrama (impairment of faith, memory, psyche and intellect).
2. Physical symptoms - fatigue, depression, taste disorders, constipation, poor digestion

Ayurvedic therapy

Katu rasam (pungent taste) ushnam (hot potency), lekhanam (erosive nature), manda nashanam (alleviating sluggishness) drugs

Bhadradarvadi kashayam – 60 ml b.d half an hour before food.

Saraswata churnam – 10 gm – b.d with honey after food.

Gorochanadi gutika – 2 b.d. after food

Panchagarya ghrtam – 10 ml h.s with milk after food.

Gomutra panam (purified cow's urine) – 30 ml at night after food

Oil for external use (Nasyam)

- Bala ashwagandha lakshadi tailam:
- Nasya (errhines) 2 drops in each nostril:
- Siro virechaneeya ganam
- Apamarga kshara tailam

Yoga basti (enema) – procedure

Yoga basti protocol.

Anuvasana basti (oil enema)–

- Dhanwantaram vasti paka – 150 ml

Niruha basti (decoction enema):

- Catwara taila -

Gomutra basti: Raja yapana basti

	Anuvasana basti (oil enema)	Niruha basti (decoction enema)
Day	1st	3rd catwara taila gomutra basti
Day	2nd	5th raja yapana basti
Day	4th	7th raja yapana basti
Day	6th	
Day	8th	

Catwara taila gomutra basti - purified cow's urine

Draya - Substance	Quantity
Makshikam - honey	120 ml
Lavanam - rock salt	15 gm
Tila Tailam with fennel seeds and camphor	120 ml
Sarshapa kalkam – paste Brassica campestris	30 gm
Dadhi mandam - whey	120 ml
Amla kaanji – processed sour gruel / vinegar	120 ml
Gomutram – purified cow's urine	60 ml
Total: Approx.	**600 ml**

Note on ayurvedic therapy with purified cow's urine:

Cow's urine has been used in ayurvedic preparations since ancient times, as mentioned in ancient sacred texts, and has long been used as an effective antiseptic against wounds and skin diseases.[116]

Diverse research has shown that cow's urine can cure diseases such as arthritis, blood pressure, psoriasis and many other diseases.

Cow's urine is also used in other areas, for example as a bio-pesticide and bio-enhancer in agriculture and is beneficial in raising honey bees. [117]

The review of the above citation concludes that formulations based on cow's urine would definitely prove to be a potential medicine that would take up the pressure on the existing use of chemicals and antibiotics. While this sounds a little unconventional to many, it could be an important step in disease management.

Enema – Raja yapana basti

Ingredients	Dose
Makshikam - honey	200 ml
Lavanam - rock salt	15 gm
Sneham - Sahacharadi oil	200 ml
Kalkam - Paste Glycyrrhizza. Glabra	30 gm
Kshira kashayam – medicated milk	300 ml
Mamsa rasam - goat meat broth	300 ml
Total: Approx	**1000 ml**

Single medications
Rudraksham - Elaeocarpus Ganitrus
Potential medicinal properties:
- Hypnotic, Sedative, anticonvulsant, antiepileptic, lowering blood pressure.

Vacha - Acorus calamus
Potential medicinal properties:
Sedative, neuroprotective, antimicrobial, anti-dyslipidemic, anti-oxidant, anticholinesterase, analgesic.

Jyotishmati - Celastrus paniculata
Potential medicinal properties:
Possess properties used to sharpen the memory.

Shanka Pushpi - Convolvulus pluricaulis
Potential medicinal properties:
Controls the production of adrenaline and cortisol in the body, thus helping to reduce anxiety and stress
Brain tonic for dementia, OCD, phobias and insomnia

Koshtam - Saussurea Lappa
Potential medicinal properties:
Anti-inflammatory, anti-cancer, liver protection, antioxidant, brain tonic[118]

Résumé

The clinical treatment methods of Ayurveda presented here as examples, generally lead to significant relief from the clinical symptoms of mental illness, such as depression, if not to complete healing.

However, lasting improvement or sustained healing will only be achieved if it is possible not only to recognize the causes or complex factors of disturbance and to respond to these with holistic treatment methods and social political measures, but also, and more importantly, to actively encourage the patient to become "aware".

This will finally lead to being ready to mobilize powers of self-healing.

In this context, at the same time leading to the final chapter, I mention a scientific study of the Professional Association of Yoga Teachers Germany e.V. with the title "Yoga in Prevention and Therapy".

At the end of this study it was found that for the effect of yoga on depression for participants in the study there was a probability in achieving a remission three times greater for patients practicing yoga, compared to patients in the study who did not practice yoga.[119]

Particularly worth noting is the effect of meditation on symptoms of depression as this increased the more meditation was practiced, during the course of the study.

In the concluding chapter, we will now explain in more detail how mental functions can be positively used and developed.

5. Ayurveda and Yoga- the magical connection of human life with the immediate environment and the universe

Here, I recall the above-mentioned reminder: to recognize one's own nature and to live accordingly is the prerequisite and goal for a fulfilled life. As long as we stay in touch with our true self - our innermost nature - our personality rests in serenity and cannot be shaken by anything.

According to ancient Indian tradition, complete well-being depends on the way gunas are pronounced. This is described in detail in many ancient scriptures, such as the Bhagavadgita or the Yogasutras.

Ayurveda and Yoga
Ayurveda uses aspects of yoga to help with the healing, proper lifestyle, and spiritual development of the individual, depending on the particular physical and mental constitution.

A true ayurvedic practitioner is therefore also a yogi. He or she controls not only the physical body, but also prana (vitality) and mind with knowledge of the subtle body and the soul. A true doctor heals through the life force, not through his own personal energy. The spirit of a true healer is attuned to the divine or inner timeless self. [120]

Here a remark seems appropriate to me, which prima facie may seem rather banal, but in my opinion with concentrated reflection a deeper meaning, if not magical meaning may be revealed.
The present has no beginning and no end!
First, let me recall the following statement by the Dalai Lama:
Man: he sacrifices his health to earn money.
Then he sacrifices his money to get his health back.
He is so focused on the future that he cannot enjoy the present.
The result is that he lives neither the future nor the present.
He lives as if he would never die and he dies as if he had never lived.

In "brevitate vitae" (shortness of life) the Stoic Lucius Annaeus Seneca expresses himself 2000 years ago [121] the future distracts from the precious moment, the past can no longer be influenced.

It is therefore the wise who know how to use the present time. "His life becomes long because he combines all times into a single one".

Here is a basic attitude of the Stoics expressed, to consider the present as the sole happiness.

Sivananda puts it this way: The present life, which is evidently revealed to you, is but a fleeting moment in eternity; so why worry about that? Better to use the moment and make the best out of it.

Live as long as there is life, and live sane and healthy according to the Gita-Dharma. Dedicate your life to the moment, and out of this connection eternal joy of life will arise.[122]

To recognize the wisdom and the voice of nature, to understand the alphabet of the elements and to live according to them is, according to the Vedic teacher (Vedacharya) Vāmadeva Śāstrī Vāmadeva, the most valuable experience of human life. [123]

Ayurveda and Yoga provide this alphabet. Ayurveda and Yoga shows the way to maintain health through a harmonious balance of body, mind and soul and yoga shows the way to transcend beyond the body consciousness.

Together Yoga and Ayurveda allow one to attain and maintain optimal health, vitality and higher awareness. This spiritual transformation is like a direct awakening that sees through the illusion of our lives (maya) and opens the door to a new vision and blissful living.

That does not mean that the world is an illusion that is now transparent. Rather, the illusion is our view of the world, when we accept the forms and structures, things, and events around us as reality, rather than realizing that they are concepts of our categorizing intellect.

Ayurveda and yoga are sources of spiritual development. Spiritual development means developing in love and training the mind to love all beings.

The first two limbs of the eight paths of Yoga (Patañjali – Ashtanga Yoga)

The yoga wisdom of Patanjali – the classical foundation of all yoga systems – teaches a spiritual perfection of man in eight stages (Ashtanga Yoga).

In the first two basic levels yoga teaches appropriate ethical behavior in social (Yama) and personal (Niyama) terms.).[124]

Primarily physical aspects are addressed by yoga asanas (predominantly resting positions), that promote suppleness and vitality, and harmonize body and mind.

Through relaxation and meditation, asanas go beyond the physical.

The more physical exercises of yoga can be juxtaposed with the physical aspect of Ayurveda – expressed in the doshas.

Patañjali, the author of the classic yoga guide (Yogasutra) about two thousand years ago, is considered the "father" of yoga. Those who follow the path of yoga experience step by step a magical connection between human life, the immediate environment and the universe.

The first five limbs (Yama, Niyama, Āsana, Prânāyāma, Pratayāhāra) are also referred to as Kriya Yoga (Practical Yoga) and the last three (Dhāranā, Dhyāna, Samādhi) as Raya Yoga (Royal yoga).
Here is the eight-limbed path at a glance:
1. Yamas – Dealing with environment
2. Niyamas – Dealing with yourself
3. Āsanas – Dealing with body
4. Prānāyāma – Dealing with breathing
5. Pratayāhāra – Dealing with the senses

6. Dhāranā – Concentration
7. Dhyāna – Meditation
8. Samādhi – The highest: Inner freedom
   (6 - 8 Samyāma – dealing with the mind)

Pratayāhāra, Dhāranā, Dhyāna, and Samādhi are considered the four inner methods and at the same time the four higher levels of yoga practice. [125]

The mind is active at this level deep into the innermost areas of the spiritual heart. However, this requires an internalization of the earlier stages of yoga - especially the ethical aspects.

These are examined in the following, because of their importance for the development of consciousness and personality development.

Sattwa, Rajas and Tamas are a kind of learning stage for Ayurveda, as already shown in the first chapter.

Likewise, the first two stages,Yama and Niyama, of the classical Ashtanga Yoga are indispensable basis for the personality development.

These ethical and moral rules of yoga, which are often overshadowed by asana in Western culture, may be the missing keys to true yogic strength and transformation, on and off the mat.

At this point it should be noted, for example, a violation of ethical aspects according to yogic view causes damage to the subtle body (aura), which subsequently has a harmful effect on the physical body.

It is striking that the first two stages of classical yoga in the practice of Western culture are usually overlooked, or are hardly mentioned, let alone paid attention. The Western understanding of yoga is more focused on the pragmatic benefits of physical muscle strengthening and therefore restricts yoga to dynamic practice of postures (asanas), breathing exercises (pranayama) and "TM" (transcendental meditation), a modified meditation form of traditional yoga.

This is regrettable because practicing yama and niyama are considered to be the most important principles in character building. [126]

The various yogic postures are recognized to have some positive effect on body, mind and soul. For example, the shoulder stand (sarvangasana) helps to cure insomnia and depression. [127]

The fish pose (Matsyasana) helps regulate mood, emotions and stress and the forward bend (Paschimottanasana) invigorates the entire nervous system.

Yoga as a body art enjoys an image in the West that promotes health.

Thus, it is not surprising that yoga practitioners usually do not consider being threatened by strokes, dislocated joints, nerve damage, paralyzed limbs, bulging eyeballs, brain damage, and lung tears, to name but a few.

William J. Broad addresses these dangers in detail in "The Science of Yoga". [128]

To make matters worse – as W. J. Broad argues – that the public silence of the gurus on the topic of injury contributes to a carefree safety attitude.

Not only the silence or the omission of a reference to potential injury hazards are to be considered but in particular also the instructions of Yoga Gurus, which they address to their students. The execution of these instructions leads in many cases to damage to health.

For example, Broad describes the Indian Yoga teacher Iyengar and founder of the yoga named after him as an incorrigible enthusiast [129] who teaches, for example, a shoulder-stand in which the chin is pressed deep into the chest and the head and chest form a right angle, whilst the body should remain in a straight line perpendicular to the ground. According to Iyengar, this exercise is said to be "one of the greatest benefits handed down to humanity by our ancient sages."

Several years ago, in Kerala, in the ayurvedic resort - where I regularly spend several weeks every year for many years - I met an attractive young lady from a rich French family. I call her Anne-Marie here. She expressed interest in my view of yoga and proudly told that she had found her guru in Iyengar and enthusiastically performed his exercises.

When I met her again back at the resort a few years later and I asked about the progress of her Iyengar yoga exercises, she openly replied that she had shelved yoga because she had a painful neck trauma with all sorts of unpleasant side effects and was still suffering with it today.

This is just one example of physical injury I have personally learned of, which has been caused by incorrect practice of yoga exercises. In other words, this behavior is a violation of the Ahimsa principle, one of the basic rules of yoga.

To address here some partially serious injuries by improperly practiced yoga exercises would go beyond the scope of the book. For those interested I recommend reading the numerous case studies of W.J. Board in the chapter "the risk of injury".

Unquestionably, positive meditation also affects the body, mind and soul. Meditation brings spiritual peace by containing the restless mind. At the physical level, meditation helps to prolong the anabolic process of growth and aid the repair of the body as well as slow down the catabolic or decaying process.

Practising Asanas, Pranayama and TM without at the same time practicing ethical principles such as truthfulness, non-violence and compassion, constitute no more than physical exercises or fitness exercises. The motivation is more the enhancement of physical performance and/or consolidating and securing material wealth rather than spiritual fulfilment in humility and contentment.

Here minds divide between East and West.

Broad reports on an experienced yogi, whose guiding principle in yoga teaching is to put less emphasis on asanas, and more on consciousness. "If you teach people asanas only, without introducing them to deeper states of consciousness, their asanas will always remain an ordeal." [130]

Not what you do with your body determines the character of an individual, but what you think and feel with your own conscious abilities. [131]

By dealing with the ethical principles of yoga, one finally becomes aware of the far-reaching and positive effects of the practical exercise of yogic ethics.

For example, in the Ethics of the Bhagavadgita, Swami Sivananda, one of the most influential spiritual teachers of the twentieth century, points out that just avoiding evil does not do much.

Rather, the simplest way to overcome the negative force of evil is to cultivate its opposite virtue. [132]

It is in the law of thought and nature that man, by sublimely or lowly thinking, can shape his character well or evilly. And further [133] just action not only attains the great purpose of life, but at the same time weakens the cosmic forces of evil by not cooperating with them, at the same time strengthening the cosmic powers of justice.

Swami Sivananda says that man creates his destiny through the power of thought. Thought sows an action and reaps a habit that ends in a character. The seed of the character gives the harvest of destiny. [134]

The following discussion of the ethical principles of yoga may clarify the profound wisdom of this ethic and the far-reaching positive effect of the practical exercise of yogic ethics.

1. Yama
Yama, the first discipline, contains rules about social behavior towards others and how to deal with the environment. This requires mindfulness and conscious interaction with fellow man.

Yama consists of five ethical principles, the realization of which requires high mental demands and daily discipline.

Ahimsa
One of the most important principles for practitioners of classical yoga is non-violence (Ahimsa). "A" in Sanskrit means "not" and the Sanskrit word "Himsa" means violence and thus Ahimsa means non-violence.

It is a rule of behavior that prohibits the killing or injuring of living beings. According to Mahatma Gandhi, the Ahimsa concept excludes both physical and mental violence, such as evil thoughts, hurtful words, hatred, dishonesty, and lies. [135]

Yoga practitioners should also avoid meat diets because eating meat violates Ahimsa's yogic principle.

According to David Frawley (Pandit Vamadeva Shastri), a distinguished author in both India and the West for his knowledge as a Vedic teacher and Padma Bushan (Lotus Order - one of the highest Indian honors) it cannot go far when the Yoga Practice is based on harming other living things. [136]

Meat food increases the animal fire in the human body and causes the tendencies of carnivorous animals to form mostly unconscious imprints and impressions (samskaras) on the human mind.

This promotes anger, desire and anxiety and other negative emotions. Frawley emphasizes that not only violence and crime but also religious intolerance has been more prevalent in the past with meat eaters. This is not only a moral but also an energetic theme for body, mind and soul both on an individual and collective level.

The renunciation of violence does not weaken, but instead develops in man a force that overcomes destructive resistance.

At this point, it should also be mentioned that in everyday dealings with Ahimsa there are very different views on how consistently non-violence should be implemented. In particular, it is debatable to what extent the use of force for personal or collective self-defense is justified.

These differences of opinion which have existed for millennia should not be referred to here, since the physiological effect of Ahimsa is thematically in the foreground of our considerations.

Thus, Paramahansa Yogananda [137] very clearly explains the deeper meaning of yoga through the Bhagavad-Gita yoga wisdom, namely to develop one's personality through self-inquiry and introspection with methods that lead to peace, inner harmony and nonviolence, to develop mental powers that recognize what promotes or hinders spiritual progress.

Swami Kriyananda [138] emphasizes that the Ahimsa principle must be understood in a subtle way, and not in a crude way. If anyone does any harm to anyone, even in the slightest way, for example, through disrespect, that person harms himself as well as the person he disrespects. [139]

The deeper meaning of Ahimsa is thus the total and complete absence not only of physical violence, but also absence of mental and spiritual violence. It is about the ability to escape or be totally free from harmful thoughts.

The Buddha and the Talmud are attributed the following findings:

The idea manifests itself as a word; the word manifests as an act, the deed becomes a habit, the habit becomes a character and the character becomes your destiny.

So pay attention to the thoughts and their ways with care. And let them arise from the love born of compassion for all living beings.

Satya
The second Yama means to truly live and deals with the issues of honesty, sincerity, faithfulness and loyalty.

Satya means to be honest, speaking the truth. To pronounce the truth requires a conscious choice of words. If the spoken truth hurts someone emotionally, it is better in the sense of Ahimsa to hold back and to be silent.

T.K.V. Desikachar [140] said: "The more truly a person speaks, the more powerful his words become."

Honesty also means not lying to oneself and admitting mistakes.

Satya thus includes honesty with others as well as sincerity towards oneself.

This has a deep meaning, because the lie breaks contact with reality and creates damaging discord in the subtle body. [141]

Why are we no longer magicians? One answer is because we break the connection to reality through lies. "Today everybody seems to lie. Bosses lie, reporters lie, politicians lie, lovers and loved lie, religious leaders lie. It seems acceptable because nobody is making a big splash about it." [142]

And further, if we "do not tear out by the root our lies, falsehoods, and our sacrificial attitude, but cover it with a spiritual facade, then science and religion may unite forever, and not a bit will change."

Asteya
'A' means not, 'steya' means steal. So the third commandment means that you do not take what you do not own; or do not steal. This means objects as well as non-physical things, such as intellectual property.

This may relate to various issues, such as the adoption of foreign texts or other representations (e.g., photos, films, sound recordings), foreign ideas (e.g., inventions), or scientific publications, copyrights.

By contrast, the flip side of stealing is to be generous, to be honest, to be affectionate.

Asteya has many aspects. Apart from the obligation to refrain from the above actions, Asteya also refers to collusion that is expressed with confidence. A breach of trust is therefore also stealing.

The hoarding of excessive wealth, not sharing one's own abilities with others, or thoughtlessly consuming natural resources can also be regarded as a form of theft.

The idea of not stealing time - the most valuable and non-renewable resource of all - is an interesting interpretation of Asteya.

Alexandra Franzen, author and columnist, adds a fitting Arabic proverb: "Open your mouth only when what you want to say is more beautiful than silence." [143]

Apart from this interpretation, some two thousand years ago Caraka mentions very pertinently in his basic work that perverse, negative, and excessive use of time, intelligence, and sensory objects is the threefold cause of both psychic and somatic disorders. [144]

Brahmacharya

Char means "move," and brahma (here in a short-form of Brahman) is "the truth." Thus, the Fourth rule of Yama means " walking in Brahman", the Supreme Being and Universal Spirit.

Brahmacharya therefore means purity in thought, in word and in deed. In order not to be distracted on the spiritual path and to protect the mind from contamination, addictive substances, sensual pleasures and sex should be avoided. [145]

Already sexual fantasies are the expression of contaminated thoughts, as also expressed in the following biblical passage of the apostle Matthew [146] "You have heard that it is said: Thou shalt not commit adultery. But I tell you, whoever looks at a woman to lust after her has already broken the marriage in the heart."

Renouncement is not a negative process such as indifference or irresponsibility, but rather in spiritual meaning the positive act of giving. [147]

Bramhacharya is also mentioned in another context.

According to the Hindu concept, Dharma is the eternal cosmic order (Sanatana Dharma) and on a human level determines Varnashrama Dharma, the social order, and is the rule of life depending on age and circumstances.

Ashrama Dharma refers to rules of moral behavior involving four stages of life, with Brahmacharya, the first of the four ages, being the stage of student life and study.

The other stages of life are Grihastya (working life, housekeeper, family formation, parenting), Vanaprastya (forest dwellers, hermit existence with maintenance of the house fire) and Samnyasa (renunciation, wandering).

The Brahmacharya period of life from childhood to the age of twenty-five focuses on education and includes the practice of chastity. [148]

During this student phase, the disciple is taught by a teacher (guru) so that he can gain spiritual liberation (moksha) at later stages of life. (Sanskrit: Moksha).[149]

Aparigraha

"Parigraha" is the greed to possess sensory objects and material things in order to enjoy them. Finally, Aparigraha, as the fifth aspect of Yama, signifies the absence of a desire for material possessions or sensory objects.

This principle is to limit possession to the necessities of life, as expressed, for example, in the following statement: "Omnia mea mecum porto" (all my possessions I carry with me).

This saying, attributed to the philosopher Bias of Priene (one of the seven sages, alongside Thales of Miletus and Solon of Athens), is meant to express that true possession is grounded in one's own abilities and qualities, and not in material things. Furthermore, Aparigraha claims not to accept gifts or rewards, if this could incur obligations or even corruption or granting of advantage, as misuse of a trust relationship would be involved.

Gifts, on the other hand, which are lovingly given out of a pure heart without any obligation associated with it, are unaffected.

Spiritual aspirants can, by practicing Nishkama Yoga, put into practice renouncing the fruits of their deeds in order to attain the highest peace or moksha.[150]

Niṣkāmakarma is the central principle of Karma Yoga and the central message of the Bhagavad Gita to follow the path to liberation through selfless action without any expectation of fruits or results.

Knowledge is better than the practice of rituals. Meditation is better than knowledge. The renunciation of the fruits of one's own deeds is better than meditation. Why? - Because the removal of expectation is immediately followed by peace. [151]

Résumé:

Deeper states of consciousness make it possible to recognize subtle connections that can be of significant meaning. Man is where his thoughts are. [152]

I call to mind again the already cited maxim, because it expresses succinctly the just mentioned:

Pay attention to your thoughts, because they will be your words,
Pay attention to your words, because they will be your actions,
Pay attention to your actions, because they will be your habits,
Pay attention to your habits, because they will be your character,
Pay attention to your character, because it will become your destiny[153]

This consciousness, which reveals itself to the outside, has its counterpart in the "inner way". The dramatist and lyric poet Christian Friedrich Hebbel emphasizes in this context man is what he thinks, what he thinks, he radiates. What he radiates, he attracts.

Man who observes and recognizes the nature of his thoughts by introspection, develops a noble character through active noble thinking and forges his destiny, he practices Ahimsa (nonviolence) and Bramacharya (purity in thought) in words and deeds, he practices Saucha (cleanliness, Hygiene).

Swami Sivananda regrets that most people do not have a sattvic background, but are hateful and jealous, and therefore failures are sure. Sattva, freed from attachment to possessions, strengthens the mind in its decision-making power, sees the unifying in diversity. The Rajasic mind, on the other hand, brings forth thoughts of the ego, becomes entangled in differences and the divisive. Tamas is usually associated with negative properties such as darkness, inertia, inhibiting (varanaka).

He, who thinks negatively, attracts what he thinks and is in resonance with the thought.

In the philosophical work of Yoga-Vasishtha, bad thoughts are regarded as the primary causes of common diseases associated with the body (Samanya). When these thoughts are lifted, the body can return to its original state and these diseases disappear. [154]

In addition to the above, ethical aspects of yoga have a psychological impact on neurological, endocrinological and immunological levels.

2. Niyama - individual self-discipline
Like Yama, Niyama belongs to the spiritual rules and also contains interesting ethical aspects, which are concerned here with dealing with oneself.

Shauca (Sauca)
This first rule of Niyama is translated as cleanliness, purity, which refers to an inner and outer aspect.

The body must be kept clean and cared for in a hygienic way, it must receive adequate nutrition, be kept in motion, so that it remains healthy, and the conditions allow its main purpose to provide mental clarity.

Inner purity is the purification of the mind from the filth of attachment, hatred, and other passions through Pratipaksha Bhavana, the method that cultivates opposing virtues. [155]

Samtosha (Santhosha)
Samtosha is a positive state of mind and means in Sanskrit contentment, modesty, joy arising from an inner serenity.

"Health is contentment, illness is discontent". This succinct definition by Caraka has already been commented on earlier on.

Satvic contentment means to take people as they are. To be more satisfied than others is a characteristic of rajasic samtosha and a lack of effort. To remain inert is an expression of tamasic samthosha.

People who are not influenced by negative or positive events, and who are also fully devoted to the Divine, are safe because they rest in the Self (Atma), not in the turmoil of the world. [156]

A serene person recognizes the world in its diversity and uniqueness. Samtosha accepts events as they arise without any expectant attitude. Even failures should be accepted, to learn from them.

Samtosha expresses a pleasant and a positive attitude to life, which, as already mentioned above in the topic "Positive psychological factors influencing the immune system", has been shown to increase the number of diverse cells involved in the immune system.

In Buddhism, equanimity (Upeksā) is one of the "four boundless states of mind" besides love, compassion and joy. In a broader sense, equanimity also includes serenity, non-attachment, non-discrimination, and letting go.

One of the purposes of the human being's expansion of consciousness is to develop the ability to recognize the unifying, instead of seeing differences between oneself and others and thus remaining in dualistic separation. [157]

Even in Western culture, the importance of a serene attitude towards well-being was highlighted more than two thousand years ago. So Lucius Annaeus Seneca was filled with serenity.

In his book "From Serenity" [158] the Roman Stoic clearly explains how one can lead one's life in harmony with oneself and one's fellow human beings. He gives timeless valid answers to this question.

One of his core sentences refers to serenity as life mastering in harmony with nature and in harmony with the infinite. Every happiness that comes from outside leaves us again. Those values, on the other hand, which are rooted within, grow and accompany us to the end.

In "Ethos of Serenity" [159], the pre-Socratic Democritus said, "to whom the inner being is well-ordered, life is also in order. Happy, whoever is modest in fortune, unfortunate, who is sullen at large."

In this context, the greeting in gilded inscription on the Holstentor, the landmark of the Hanseatic city of Lübeck, is cited again: "Concordia domi foris pax", which means like "inside concord – outside peace".

In the state of Swasthya our personality remains in serenity and cannot be shaken by anything. Ayurveda considers the ability to recognize one's own nature and to stay in contact with our true self as a prerequisite and goal for a fulfilled life.

Tapas

Tapas is the bid to keep the body healthy by stoking the "inner embers". This creates the basis for achieving mental clarity.

For example, Āsanas and Prânāyāma are used to heat the body and thus release impurities in the excretion, skin and respiration.

As a result, the body can cleanse itself of toxins in the food and also of ordinary "slags", such as toxic end products of protein degradation.

In addition, the above-mentioned yoga exercises help to gain mental clarity, as they completely reduce accumulated "psycho-rubbish".

Svādhāya (Svadhyaya)

"Sva" in Sanskrit means "self" and "adhyaya" means "exploration". Svadhyaya therefore means to explore the self.

The commandment of self-inquiry requires reflection of the ego - to recognize oneself, to become conscious, to be able to criticize oneself.

I have already mentioned the meaning of "Know thyself". In the search for an answer to the question who am I, in the sense of Svādhāya, one focuses on the highest self.

To be inspired, one should study texts with a spiritual, philosophical or religious background.

Ishvara-Pranidhana (Ishvarapranidhana)

The fifth commandment is translated as "turning to God."

As a synonym for God, this can mean, among other things, creation, universal spirit, cosmic law, transcendent reality.

Ishvara-Pranidhāna also means freeing oneself from fears and doubts and feeling secure in the trust of God or even basic trust.

This basic trust is the basis for healthy self-confidence and happy life. It shapes the character of a child as early as the first years of life, provides emotional security and is the basis for the development of self-esteem, trust in a partnership, friendship and in general a fearless debate with the social world.

The ability to free oneself from attachments, prejudices and similar constraints requires abandoning expectations, letting go and letting things happen.

It is about the divine will to acknowledge the cosmic order (Sanatana Dharma) or the true nature of the Universe and to cognitively align one's own life-style accordingly.

It is necessary to put aside his own will, as expressed in the Lord's Prayer – the most important prayer of Christianity – by "Thy will be done, as in heaven, on earth" (fiat voluntas tua, sicut in caelo, et in terra).

In a time marked by individualism and self-determination thinking, where one's own selfish will (ego) is the yardstick of volition and action, little understanding is offered to this verse.
The living experience on earth, however, should be fulfilled by the spiritual principle.
Letting go of everyday thoughts, for example by practicing yoga exercises and especially meditation, leads to more concentration on tasks and duties that can be better fulfilled.

Résumé:
Niyama as a personal discipline and at the same time ethics in personal life style and Yama, ethics in dealing with others are not rigid rules, but wisdom and advice for a peaceful way of life.

Implementing the recommendations of Niyama and Yama into one's own life helps to clarify the mind, and to achieve spiritual development and a happy and successful life.

Satisfaction, modesty, purity of thought, trust, serenity, enjoying the moment are aspects that an infant - not yet conditioned by the school and parents' home – experiences naturally without fear.

This attitude is usually difficult for adults as they are plagued by worries about the future, fears of the present, and melancholy evoked by memories of the past.

A child trusts indiscriminately and lives happily "in the here and now". This is what the biblical passage points to: "Unless you convert and become like children, you will not enter into the kingdom of heaven."(*Matthew 18:3*) and "Let the little ones come to me, and do not keep them away: for of such is the kingdom of heaven." (*Matthew 19:14*)

This reversal to basic trust reveals the ethical principles of Yama and Niyama, such as:
Ahimsa, the renunciation of any violence
Satya, to live honestly
Bramacharya, a life in harmony with Sanatana Dharma (the eternal cosmic order) and Varnashrama Dharma (social order)
Aparigraha, freedom from attachments,
Shauca, purity in thought, word and deed
Samtosha, simple needs, modesty, humility
Tapas, create mental clarity
Svādhāya, self-analysis, self-knowledge
Ishvara-Pranidhāna, basic trust, freedom from fears, doubts and worries

Note on ethics related to the ethical aspect of yoga
The current 14th Dalai Lama, known for his peaceful work throughout the world, encourages a return to an ethics inherent in all human beings as the basis for a just, respectful and peaceful coexistence beyond religion with his appeal "Ethics is more important than religion". Only a return to this ethic can solve the deep conflicts and secure the future of humanity. It is not religions that will give the answer, but the rootedness of man in ethics overcoming differences.

Although the ideas of the spiritual leader of Tibetan Buddhism have so far been denied political implementation, this courageous appeal of the humble and, through his charisma, impressive person has increased the awareness of many people around the world as strengthening for a fairer togetherness is felt.

Many friends and acquaintances have spoken to me in admiration of what they believe to be the encouraging call of the spiritual leader of the Tibetans.

To my reply that I cannot see any contradiction between religion and ethics, at least not from a Christian point of view, my interlocutors react with incomprehension: One cannot turn the wheel of history and therefore must pragmatically approach today's problems. That which seems feasible according to the practical conditions should be implemented.

That sounds plausible, but it causes me to say something like this:

Right at the beginning of his remarks in "Ethics is more important than religion," the Dalai Lama emphasizes that religions were often abused to enforce political or economic interests.

I interpret that as an admission. It is not religion which is incapable of ensuring peaceful co-existence among human beings, but the misappropriation of the very essence of religion by mankind.

For example, the very essence not only of the Christian religion is the love of God and of every human being.

"God is love, and he who remains in love abides in God, and God abides in him". (1 John 4: 16b) "Fear is not in love, but complete love drives out fear; because fear is painful. But he that is afraid is not wholly in love "(1 John 4:18).

Religion captures the inner life, heart and soul.

Ethics deals with the evaluation of human action and, together with legal, political and social philosophy, is understood as a practical philosophy. (160)

The secularized form of religion reduces love to ethics.

It is the binding power of love that allows the dignity and freedom of the other person in the community to unfold, and not a man-made hierarchy, organization or behavioral pattern devised by the human mind.

"We need to discover the power of love and if we do that, we will be able to create a new world out of this old world. Love is the only way," preached Michael Bruce

Curry, Chief Bishop of the Episcopal Church of America, during the wedding ceremony of Prince Harry and Duchess Meghan.

Later, Curry reaffirmed that their love for each other has brought us together, even if only for a brief moment. It has allowed us to cross the boundaries of nationality, race and politics.

Their love has helped change our dealings with others, even if it was only for a moment, it became clear that this love could help us change the world and make it a little better.

Love is the biggest growth impulse ever (Bruce Lipton) [161]

"There is only one religion, the religion of love" (Swami Sivananda).

Epilogue

On the hike along the path of ayurvedic wisdom, having arrived at this point, may a review and a forward view let us behave more consciously and responsibly, be more considerate with our fellow human beings and be more gentle with the environment in which we live and through which we can live.

Reflectively, may we linger in a scrutinizing and thoughtful way and create an inner picture of the future in the vision.

Medicine without soul is "dead medicine", medicine without morality and ethics is "irresponsible medicine", medicine without religion is "loveless medicine".

Man, who can split atoms and does not love, becomes a monster.

Mbih Jerome Tosam sees complementary forms in philosophy and medicine. Philosophy is the search for the truth and medicine is the search for health. Both complement each other and are committed to improving human well-being.

Hontschik affirms that medical art consists in treating the sick as a subject, as a living being.

"Psychosomatic means that body and soul are two inseparable aspects of the human being, distinguished only for methodological reasons or for better understanding.

Mental problems do not cause physical disorders: they are!

Psycho-Neuro-Endocrino-Sozio-Immunology sees diseases of the body and diseases of the mind not as separate manifestations of physical being, but connected by complex interactions.

Ayurveda is a holistic medicine that considers the body, mind and soul of the human being as a unity.

Ayurvedic medicine recognizes a unity in microcosm and macrocosm. Building blocks of the universe are five elements (Mahabhoutas). All manifestations of nature – including man in his physical manifestation and psychic tendencies – are composed of the five elements earth, water, fire, air and ether (space).

The different composition of the elements is decisive for a more material manifestation or more subtle (mental) manifestation.

"God rests in stone, sleeps in the plant, dreams in the animal and awakens in the human being" [162]

As long as we are in contact with our true self, our innermost nature, we are in a balanced and powerful state at all levels of our personality.

Resilient in the basic trust or in the words of the resistance fighter Dietrich Bonhoeffer, "from good powers wonderfully safe, we confidently await what may come".

In the dialogue "The Ending of Time" [163], quantum physicist David Bohm and the philosopher Jiddu Krishnamurti express that humanity can fundamentally change as long as a transformation is made from the narrow and particular interests of the individual to the common good, which springs from a deeper purity of compassion, love, and intelligence beyond thought and time

To recognize one's own nature, to live by selfless love in harmonious community is the prerequisite and the goal for a long, healthy and fulfilling life.

FINIS

References

(1)   Vasant Lad,Textbook of Ayurveda, Volume Three: General Principles of Management and Treatment Vasant Lad,The Complete Book of Ayurvedic Home Remedies: Based on the Timeless Wisdom of India's 5,000-Year-Old Medical System Paperback – April 6, 1999
Vasant Lad, Ayurveda: The Science of Self Healing: A Practical Guide Paperback – 1985
Maya Tiwari, Ayurveda Secrets of Healing Paperback – August 23, 1995
David Frawley, Ayurvedic Healing: A Comprehensive Guide Paperback – April 23, 2001
David Frawley, Ayurveda and the Mind: The Healing of Consciousness Paperback – March 21, 1997

(2)   Jorge Bucay "Das Buch der Weisheit" Wege zum Wissen, S. Fischer Verlag, 2015 ISBN 978-3-596-19797-2, S.23

(3)   The Dance of Shiva, Ananda Coomaraswamy)

(4)   Sri Ramana Maharshi (Über das Selbst, Vierzig Verse, S.5,Drei Eichen Verlag,1996, ISBN 978-3-7699-0569-4)

(5)   (Quelle: www.hermetik.ch)

(6)   http://www.allesistenergie.net/der-makrokosmos-ist-ein-abbild-des-mikrokosmos-und-umgekehrt-fraktalitaet-entsprechung-strukturel

(7)   http://www.phyx.at/mikrokosmos/

(8)   https://www.nmz.de/online/die-welt-ist-klang-swr2-praesentiert-joachim-ernst-berendts-kultsendung-von-1981

(9)   1.Mose 1.1, Johannes 17.5, Offenbarung 19.13

(10) 1.Korinther 8.6,, Kolosser 1.16-17, Hebräer1.2

(11) Johannes 8.12

(12) Johannes 3.19

(13) Nada Brahma: Die Welt ist Klang (suhrkamp taschenbuch) Taschenbuch – 2007

(14) https://wiki.yoga-vidya.de/Om

(15) Professor Klaus Fessmann , Pianist, Komponist und Klangkünstler (s. E-mail 23.02.2018)

(16) Armin Risi, Ein spirituell-philosophisches Handbuch1. Auflage September 2004, 4. Auflage 2016, gebunden, 504 Seiten,ISBN 978-3-906347-62-2.

(17) Es werde Licht: Die Einheit von Geist und Materie in der Quantenphysik | Frido Mann, Christine Mann | ISBN: 9783103972450.

(18) http://www.weisheitsrichinmoys.com/themen/licht

(19) 15. Kap, Vers 15)   Jack Hawley, Bhagavadgita 191.

(20) Bhagavadgita, Kap 8

(21) Johann Wolfgang von Goethe, Sämtliche Werke in 18 Bänden, Band 1: Sämtliche Gedichte. Artemis, Zürich 1950, S. 514.

(21a) Dr. K.V. Dilipkumar: Clincal Yoga & Ayurveda, The Chaukamba Ayurvijnan Studies 101, 2010 Publishers: Chaukamba Sanskrit Pratishthan, 38 U.A.Bungalow Road, Jawahar Nagar, Delhi 11007

(22) Martin G. Weiß: Die Auflösung der menschlichen Natur. In: Martin G. Weiß (Hrsg.): Bios und Zoë. Suhrkamp, Frankfurt a.M. 2009, ISBN 978-3-518-29499-4, S.46.

(23) Katha Upanishad (Vers 3, 10)

(24) Gregory Bassham: Von den Veden bis zum neuen Atheismus, DAS PHILOSOPHIEBUCH: 250 Meilensteine in der Geschichte der Philosophie, 2018, S.12 (Die Veden),ISBN: 978-90-8998-944-4

(25) Klaus-Rupprecht Wasmuht Ayurveda und Gesundheit –Mehr Freude durch bewusstes Leben - Vier Beiträge für ein gesundes und erfülltes Leben aus ayurvedischer Sicht, Books on Demand GmbH, Norderstedt, 2012, ISBN 978-3-8448-2032-4

(26) What Is Life? The Physical Aspect of the Living Cell, Erwin Schrödinger Publication Date 1944, 1948 Edition ISBN 0-521-42708-8

(27) Science and Humanism: Physics in Our Time (SCIENCE, PHYSICS, PHILOSOPHY) Hardcover – 1961, CAMBRIDGE UNIVERSITY PRESS

(28) https://de. wikipedia.org/wiki/Integraler Yoga

(29) Otto Wolff: Der Integrale Yoga S. 74 (Übersetzung aus Letters of Sri Aurobindo S. 282 f.)

(30) Ayurvedic Healing, A Comprehensive Guide, 2nd Revised and Enlarged Edition, Copyright © 2000 by David Frawley, ISBN 0-914955-97-7

(31) http://www.gesundheitlicheaufklaerung.de/der-geist-ist-staerker-als-die-gene

(32) Intelligente Zellen – Wie Erfahrungen unsere Gene steuern, Bruce Lipton, Koha Verlag, ISBN 978-3-936862-88-1

(33) Sivananda All about Hinduism, S.185

(34) Rudolf Virchow: Rede auf dem XI. internationalen medizinischen Kongress in Rom 1894

(35) H C Crick, "Was die Seele wirklich ist-Die naturwissenschaftliche Erforschung des Bewußtseins Rowohlt, 1997, ISBN 3-499-60257-1 (englisches Original: The astonishing hypothesis: the scientific search for the soul, Scribner 1995)

(36) Louis Cozolino: Die Neurobiologie menschlicher Beziehungen, VAK Verlags GmbH, Kirchzarten bei Freiburg, 2007, S.14, ISBN 978-3-86731-001-7; Titel der amerikanischen Originalausgabe: The Neuroscience of Human Relationship

(37) Karl Wimmer: Was ist die Seele? Eine alte Frage neu gestellt, S.7, Karl Wimmer & Partner, Netzwerk für balancierte Entwicklung, http://www.wimmer-partner.at/pdf.dateien/seele.pdf

(38) Karl Wimmer: Was ist die Seele?, ebenda, S.8

(39) Stefan Zweig: Die Heilung durch den Geist, Fischer Taschenbuchverlag, Frankfurt am Main, 1998, S.13, ISBN 3-596-22300-8)

(40) Stefan Zweig: Die Heilung durch den Geist, ebenda,S.301

(41) Mbih Jerome Tosam: The Role of Philosophy in Modern Medicine, Open Journal of Philosophy Vol.04 No.01(2014), Article ID:43303, Department of Philosophy, Higher Teacher Training College (HTTC)Bambili, University of Bamenda, Bamenda, Cameroon, http://file.scirp.org/Html/11-1650321_43303.htm

(42) Dr. Bernd Hontschik, Körper, Seele Mensch – Versuch über die Kunst des Heilens, Suhrkamp, ISBN: 978-3-518-45818-1

(43) Dr. Remya Krishnan:Evidence Based Ayurveda & Rational Prescribing,2012 Vision Grafix, Trivandrum - 695012

(44) Pietschmann, Die erweiterte einheitliche Quantenfeldtheorie von Burkhard Heim, Wolfgang Ludwig – Innsbruck: Resch, 1998 (Grenzfragen<)>: 17, ISBN 3-85382-963-8

(45) Dr. V.Coleman, Die moderne Medizin ist keine Wissenschaft, https:///naturepower.de/vitalstofff-journal/fakten-widerreden/medizinbetrieb/die-moderne-medizin-ist-keine-wissenschaft

(46) Dr. Issac Mathai: Holistic Healing- A doctor`s guide to rediscovering health and happiness, naturally, 2014, S.68 /s.84, ISBN 978-935029-093-4

(47) David Frawley, Vom Geist des Ayurveda: Therapien für den Geist, Yogische ganzheitliche Medizin und ayurvedische Psychologie, Windpferd Verlag, S.120

(48) J.Krishnamurti: Wie willst Du leben?, S.224 (Originaltext: What are you

doing with your life?), Arbor Verlag, Freiamt im Schwarzwald, 2006, ISBN 3-936855-27-7

(49) https://de.wikipedia.org/wiki/Psychosomatik

(50) Axel Schweickhardt, Kurt Fritzsche, Michael Wirsching: Psychosomatische Medizin und Psychotherapie (Springer Lehrbuch) S. 5 und 7, Heidelberg 2005, ISBN 3540218777

(51) Psychoneuroimmunology 4th Edition, Editor-in-Chiefs: Robert Ader, 2006,ISBN: 9780120885763

(52) Lown, Bernard, Die verlorene Kunst des Heilens: Anstiftung zum Umdenken, Schattauer Verlag – 1. Nachdruck 2008, ISBN:978-3-7945-2347-4

(53) Louis Cozolino, ebenda S. 20

(54) http://www.planet-wissen. de/gesellschaft/medizin/psychosomatik/pwiedernoceboefffekt100.html

(55) Walter Feichtinger http://www.meduniwien.ac.at/med_audiovisiuals/Seminare/Powerpoint /SymbolischesHeilen-I/VooDoo%20Death.pdf

(56) Walter Feichtinger, ebenda

(57) R.Adler, N.Cohen: Behaviorally conditioned immunsupression. In: Psychosomatic medicine, Band 37, Nummer 4´, 1975, S.333-340, ISSN 0033-3174. PMID 1162023

(58) https://de.wikipedia.org/wiki/Psychoneuroimmunologie

(59) Christian Schubert: *Psychoneuroimmunologie und Psychotherapie*. Schattauer Verlag, 2011, ISBN 978-3-7945-2700-7, S. 116.

(60) Taylor, E.S. & Brown, J.D. (1988). Illusion and well-being: A social psychological perspective on mental health. In: *Psychological Bulletin, 103 (2)*, 193-210.

(61) J. E. Milram, J. L. Richardson, G. Marks, C. A. Kemper, A. J. McCutchan: *The roles of dispositional optimism and pessimism in HIV disease progression*. In: *Psychol Helth*. 2004; 19, S. 167–181.

(62) T. Miyazaki, S. Ishilkawa, A. Natata u. a.: *Association between perceived social support and Th1 dominance*. In: *Biol Psychology*. 2005; 70, S. 30–37

(63) Louis Cozolino: Neurologie menschlicher Beziehungen,2006, ISBN 978-0-393-70454-9, VAK Verlags GmbH, Kirchzarten bei Freiburg,

(64) Louis Cozolino: Neurologie menschlicher Beziehungen, ebenda

(65) Der Crash ist die Lösung", Matthias Weik & Marc Friedrich, Bastel Lübbe Taschenbuch, Band 60858,2015, ISBN 978-3-404-60858-4

(66) C.G.Jung: Zugang zum Unbewussten; Die menschliche Seele in: Der

Mensch und seine Symbole, 8. Auflage der Sonderausgabe 1985, ISBN 3-530-56501-4 und https://zitatezumnachdenken.com/carl-gustav-jun

(67) Jesaja 42,8

(68) Exodus 20,3

(69) http://namastetruckee.com/namaste-defined

(70) Jack Hawley,Bhagavad Gita, Der Gesang Gottes, Eine zeitgemäße Version für westliche Leser, Goldmann Arkana, 4.Auflage 2002, ISBN 078-3-442-21607-9, S.109ff

(71) Jack Hawley, Bhagavadgita, ebenda

(72) Fritjof Capra: The turning Point; Scienc0e , Sovciety, and the Rising Culture, 1984 ISBN-13:978-0553345728

(72a) Sri Raman Maharshi:Über das Selbst – vierzig Verse, kommentiert und erläutert von Mata Satymayi, autorisierte Übertragung aus "The collected works of Ramana Maharshi",Drei Eichen Verlag Seite 23, 3. Auflage 2007, ISBN 978-3-7699-0569-4

(73) Friedrich von Schiller "Über die ästhetische Erziehung des Menschen",8. Brief

(74) Dr. David Frawley: Vom Geist des Ayurveda. Therapien für den Geist, Yogische ganzheitliche Medizin und ayurvedische Psychologie,, Windpferd Verlag, aus dem Amerikanischen von Rita Penny, 2. Auflage 2003, ISBN 3-89385-304-9, S.122ff

(75) C. G. Jung: *Gesammelte Werke*. 7, 266, 404.

(76) M.-L. von Franz, Der Individuationsprozess in C.G.Jung. "Der Mensch und seine Symbole", 8. Auflage der Sonderausgabe . 1985, Walter Verlag AG, Olten, S. 162, ISBN 3-530-56501-6

(77) https://vedanta-yoga.de/bhagavad-gita-verse-6-1-6-9-innere-entsagung

(78) C. G. Jung: Die Beziehungen zwischen dem Ich und dem Unbewußten. Zweiter Teil: Die Individuation. 4. Auflage. dtv, München, S. 116.

(79) Aristoteles: Metaphysik. Ins Deutsche übertragen von Adolf Lasson. Jena 1907, S. 129

(80) Charaka Samhitā,(Text with English Translat on)P.V. Sharma, Chaukhambha Orientalia, Varanasi, India, 2007, Volume I, Section of Fundamentals, Chapter IX,4, ISBN81-7637-012-6

(81) https://www.berliner-zeitung.de/26228800 ©2018

(82) Social Justice in the EU – Index Report 2017, Social Inclusion Monitor Europe, Daniel Schwaad-Tischler, Cristof Schiller, Sascha Matthias Heller, Nina Siemer, Bertelsmann Verlag

(83)   https://www.transparency.org/cpi2014/results

(84)   Meik Wiking, "The Little Book of Hygge, the Danish way to live well",Pinguin Random House, UK 2016, S.62, ISBN:978-0-241-28391-2

(85)   Meik Wiking, "The little Book of Lykke, The Danish Search for the World`s Happiest People" Pinguin Random House, UK 2017, S.1302, ISBN: 978-0-241-30201-9

(86)   http://ec.europa.eu/eurostat/statistics-explained/images/5/5f/Causes_of_death_standardised_death_rate%2C-2014_(per_ 100_000-inhabitants)

(87)   Daniel Everett: Das glücklichste Volk, Sieben Jahre bei den Pirahã-Indianern am Amazonas. DVA Sachbuch, München 2012, ISBN 978-3-570-55167-7

(88)   Jack Hawley (Hrsg.) Bhagavadgita – Der Gesang Gottes,Eine zeitgemäße Version für westliche Leser, Aus dem Amerikanischen von Peter Kobbe, Goldmann ARKANA, München, 2002, ISBN 978-3-442-21607-9. 2. Kapitel, S.53

(89)   Jack Hawley,ebenda S 49

(90)   Jack Hawley,ebenda S 40

(91)   Charaka Samhitã,(Text with English Translation) P.V. Sharma, Chaukhambha Orientalia, Varanasi, India, 2007, Volume I, 4. Section on the study of human body: Chapter I, 152/153, ISBN81-7637-012-6

(92)   Psychotherapie in Deutschland- Versorgung, Zufriedenheit, Klima- 2011, Dossier zur Online Studie von Pro Psychotherapie e.V. https://www.therapie.de/fileadmin/dokumente/pi/Dossier_Umfrageergebnisse_zu_Psychother-apie_in_Deutschland_2011_therapie.de.pdf

(93)   Frawley ebenda, S.197

(94)   Sushruta Samhita Sutrasthana, 15/41)

(95)   -Psychyrembel, 2004

(96)   http://www.mind-control-news.de/seiten/display/who-definition-gesundheit/

(97)   Klaus Hurrelmann: Gesundheitssoziolgie, eine Einführung in sozialwissenschaftliche Theorien, von Krankheitsprävention und Gesundheitsförderung, Reihe Grundlagentexte Soziologie, Verlag Juventa, ISBN 978-37799-1483-9

(98)   Csikszentmihalyi, M. (1990). Flow: The Psychology of Optimal Experience. New York: Harper and Row. ISBN 0-06-092043-2

(99)   https://www.golfdigest.com/story/myshot_gd0210

(100) Hebräer 12,27

(101) Csikszentmihalyi, M. (1990). Flow: The Psychology of Optimal Experience. New York: Harper and Row. ISBN 0-06-092043-2

(102) http://www.chopra.com/article/what-oneness#sm.0001ye1y2hinffduu3y-1cywv9c4e4 By Roger Gabriel (Raghavanand)

(103) http://www.ayurindus.com/ayurveda/definition-of-health/

(104) THE BHAGAVADGITA, ebenda, XII, S.77.

(105) Ashtanga Hrdayam, Sutra Sthana, Srimad Vagbhata, in der Übersetzung von Hendrik Wiethase, Wiethase Verlag, 2006, XI, 6-8, ISBN 3-937632-43-4

(106) https://de.scribd.com/doc/30500784/Manasa-roga

(107) Unmada-Insanity": Ayurvedic Understanding and Management" Dr. MS Krishnamurthy MD (Ayu), PhD (Ayu) https://easyayurveda.com/2014/04/18/unmada-insanity-ayurvedic-understanding-management

(108) Worshipping the Fire: Kama (Lust) - Paramahansa Yogananda http://worshippingthefire.blogspot.com/2009/05/kama-lust-paramahansa-yogananda.html

(109) Commentaries of the Four Authorized Vaisnava Sampradayas / Sridhara Swami's Commentary http://www.bhagavad-gita.org/Gita/verse-03-37.html

(110) https://en.wikipedia.org/wiki/Arishadvargas

(111) Commentary by Sri A.C. Bhaktivedanta Swami Prabhupada of Gaudiya Sampradaya: https://www.bhagavad-gita.us/bhagavad-gita-18-73/

(112) http://www.yoga-vidya.de/de/artikel/sivananda/bezwingung_eifersucht.html und https://www.yoga-vidya.de/yoga-buch/sivananda/samadhi-yoga/kapitel-v-negative-eigenschaften/4-hass-und-eifersucht/

(113) http://www.der-innere-weg.de/der-innere-weg/schatztruhe/achte-auf-deine-gedanken/ (mit folgendem Hinweis: Weisheit aus unbekannter Quelle; Charles Reade hat zu seiner Verbreitung verholfen; wird einem Sprichwort aus China zugeschrieben – oft auch fälschlicherweise dem Talmud)

(114) http://www.ramakrishna.de/vedanta/bhagavad-gita16.php

(115) Ayurvedic Management of Manic-Depressive Disorder, Dr. L Mahadevan B.A.M.S., M.D. Dr. Y Mahadeva Iyer's Hospital, Derisanamcope,Tamil Nadu, Indien (Sript)

(116) https://www.timesnownews.com/health/article/seven-health-benefits-of-cow-urine-that-will-surprise-you/73375

(117) "diversifizierte Verwendungen von Kuhurin", veröffentlicht im Interna-

tional Journal of Pharmacy and Pharmaceutical Sciences Vol. 6, Issue 3, 2014, ISSN 0975-1491

(118) Ayurvedic management of Manic-Depressive disorder (Script),ebenda

(119) https://www.yoga.de/site/assets/files/1441/yoga_in_praevention_ und-therapie5-2015.pdf

(120) David Frawley, Yoga & Ayurveda, Self-Healing and Self-Realization, S 172/173 Lotus Press, P.O. Nox 325, Twin Lakes, Wisconsin 53181, ISBN 0-9-81-014955

(121) L.Annaeus Seneca: De brevitate vitae – Von der Kürze des Lebens : Lateinisch /Deutsch übersetzt und herausgegeben von Marion Giebel, Reclam 2008, S.55ff ISBN 978-3-15-018545-2…

(122) Sivananda Ethics of the Gita S42

(123) David Frawley (Vāmadeva Śāstrī), Yoga und Ayurveda, Self-Healing and Self-Realization, ebenda

(124) Sukadev Volker Bretz, Die Yogaweisheit des Patanjali für Menschen von heute, 3. Auflage 2008, Verlag Via Nova, ISBN 978-3-928632-81-2,

(125) David Frawley: Vom Geist des Ayurveda, ebenda S.238–

(126) Dr. Mangalagowri V. Rao "The Essence of Yoga" CHAUKAMBHA ORIENTALIA, Varanasi, First Edition 2011, S.212, ISBN 978-81-7637-250-3

(127) The Sivananda Yoga Training Manual, Sivananda Yoga Vedanta Centre, 1991, 673, 8th Avenue, Val Morin, Quebec, Canada, JOT 2RO.

(128) William J. Broad, The Science of Yoga, The Risks and the Rewards (aus dem Amerikanischen von Maren Klostermann), Herder GmbH, Freiburg i.Br. 2013, 161ff, ISBN 978-3-451-30685-3

(129) William J. Broad, The Science of Yoga, ebenda, S 117

(130) William J. Broad, ebenda S 167)

(131) Ethics of the Bhagavadgita , Swami Sivananda, The Divine Life Society, P.O. Shivanandanagar 249 192, Ditt. Tehri-Garhwal, U.P. Himalayas, India , 1995, S. 26, ISBN81-7052-099-1

(132) Ethics of the Bhagavadgita, Swami Sivananda, ebenda, S 102)

(133) Ethics of the Bhagavadgita, Swami Sivananda, ebenda, Seite 173)

(134) Swami Sivananda, "die Kraft der Gedanken", Mangalam Books, Sivananda Yoga Vedanta Zentrum München, 2003, S.28, ISBN 3-922477-09-7

(135) Koshelya Walli: *The Conception of Ahimsa in Indian Thought*, Varanasi 1974, S. XXII–XLVII; William Borman: *Gandhi and Non-Violence*, Albany 1986, S. 11

(136) David Frawley, Yoga & Ayurveda, Self-Healing and Self-Realization, S

172/173 Lotus Press, P.O. Nox 325, Twin Lakes, Wisconsin 53181, ISBN 0-9-81-014955

(137) Yogananda, Paramahansa, Der Yoga der Bhagavadgita, Eine Einführung in die universale indische Wissenschaft der Gottverwirklichung, Self Realization Fellowship, 2008 , S. 224, ISBN 978-0-87612-034-7

(138) https://www.ananda.org/yogapedia/ahimsa/a b The Art and Science of Raja Yoga, Swami Kriyananda. Step 4, "Yama"

(139) https://www.mindbodygreen.com/0-4954/What-Does-Ahimsa-Really-Mean.html

(140) https://yoga-cara.de/wp-content/uploads/Der-Achtgliedrige-Pfad.pdf

(141) William Arntz, Betsy Chasse, Mark Vicente: Bleep, An der Schnittstelle von Spiritualität und Wissenschaft, VAK Verlags GmbH, Kirchzarten, 3. Aufl. 2006 ISBN 13-978-3-935767-84-2.1

(142) William Arntz, Betsy Chasse, Mark Vicente: Bleep,, ebenda

(143) http://www.alexandrafranzen.com/2013/03/15/how-to-practice-asteya/

(144) Charaka Samhitã,(Text with English Transltion) P.V. Sharma, Chaukhambha Orientalia, Varanasi, India, 2007, Volume I, Section on Fundamentals, Chapter I, 54 ISBN81-7637-012-6

(145) Bhagavad Gita, der Gesang Gottes, Jack Hawley, ebenda,

(146) Matth. 5,27/28

(147) Bhagavad Gita, der Gesang Gottes, Jack Hawley, ebenda, S.209

(148) RK Sharma (1999), Indian Society, Institutions and Change, ISBN 978-8171566655, S.28

(149) Georg Feuerstein, The Encyclopedia of Yoga and Tantra, Shambhala Publications, ISBN 978-1590308790, 2011, page 76, und W.J. Johnson (2009), "The chaste and celibate state of a student of the Veda", Oxford Dictionary of Hinduism, Oxford University Press, ISBN 978-2713223273,S 62

(150) Bhagavadgita 13,7 Kommentar von Swami Sivananda in: The Bhagavad Gita,, Eleventh edition 2003, The Divine Life Trust Society, , published and printed by Swami Jivanmuktananda at the Yoga-Vedanta Forest Academy Press, P.o. Shivanandanagar, Distt. Tehri-Garhwal, Uttaranchal, Himalayas, India, ISBN 81-7052-000-2

(151) Bhagavad Gita, der Gesang Gottes Eine zeitgemäße Version für westliche Leser, Kapitel XII, Vers 12, S.160, Jack Hawley (Hrsg.)   Aus dem Amerikanischen von Peter Kobbe,, Goldmann Arkana4. Auflage 2002, ISBN 978-3-442-21607

(152) Bhagavad Gita, der Gesang Gottes, ebenda, Kapitel XII, Vers 8, S.159

(153) Weisheit aus unbekannter Quelle; Charles Reade hat zu seiner Verbreitung verholfen; wird einem Sprichwort aus China – (oft auch fälschlicherweise dem Talmud)zugesc hrieben

(154) Dilipkumar, Dr. K.V. Dilipkumar: Clincal Yoga & Ayurveda, The Chaukamba Ayurvijnan Studies S.112, 2010 Publishers: Chaukamba Sanskrit Pratishthan, 38 U.A.Bungalow Road, Jawahar Nagar, Delhi 11007

(155) Bhagavadgita 13,7 Kommentar von Swami Sivananda in: The Bhagavad Gita,, Eleventh edition 2003, The Divine Life Trust Society, , published and printed by Swami Jivanmuktananda at the Yoga-Vedanta Forest Acadenmy Press, P.o. Shivanandanagar, Distt. Tehri-Garhwal, Uttaranchal, Himalayas, India, ISBN 81-7052-000-2

(156) Bhagavad Gita, der Gesang Gottes, ebenda, Kapitel II, 56,57,S.53 und Kapitel XII,Vers 8

(157) Das Herz von Buddhas Lehre Leiden verwandeln - die Praxis des glücklichen Lebens von Thich Nhat Hanh (Autor)   Verlag Herder, 8. Auflage 2016, ISBN: 978-3-451-05412-9

(158) Seneca: De brevitate vitae – Von der Kürze des Lebens, übersetzt und herausgegeben von Marion Giebel, Reclams Universalbibliothek Nr.18545, 2008, ISBN 978-3-15-018545-2

(159) Kleine Philosophie der Faulheit, David Dilmaghani und Nassima Sahraoui, Fischer Verlag,| ISBN: 978-3-596-90496-9

(160) https://de.wikipedia.org/wiki/Ethik

(161) https://www.lifeandlove.de/bruce-lipton-intelligente-zellen.htm

(162) Rabindranath Tagore, 1861–1941;Indische Weisheiten für jeden Tag,2011 (Fischer Klassik, Axel Monte, Herausgeber, Übersetzer)

(163) The Ending of Time: Where Philosophy and Physics Meet , J.Krisnamurti & David Bohm, 2014, Imprint HarperOne, ISBN:9780062360977; ISBN 10:0062360973

Vita

Klaus-Rupprecht Wasmuht, born April 10, 1941 in Dortmund, Diploma (Abitur) in 1962 at the Humboldt Gymnasium, Dortmund. Then half-year study trip through South America.

First contacts with healing methods of indigenous people, especially shamanism of the Bororo Indians on the Rio Jauqoara,Mato Grosso, Brazil.

1962 - 1964 military service with the medical force of the Bundeswehr (Federal Armed Forces), among others in the military hospital, Coblenz and in the medical academy, Munich. Training in first aid and nursing. Graduation with the rank of lieutenant of the reserve, after further military exercises in the Mobile Army Surgical Hospital promoted to the rank of first lieutenant of the reserve.

1964 - 1966 private education as a naturopath at Otto Riede, Munich with conclusion and receipt of the certificate of appointment from the health authority of the City of Munich.

1964 - 1968 Studied business administration at the Maximilian University of Munich and Wilhelms University in Muenster i.W.; completed with diploma in business administration.

1969 - 1973 research associate at the Ruhr University Bochum; married, father of four children.

1974 - 1980 Klöckner & Co. KGaA, Duisburg, first as assistant director of finance,

Gold medal with the team Klöckner & Co KGaA at the German business plan game 1975, organizer: University seminar Cologne and the business newspaper Handelsblatt.

1980 - 1992 Finance Director of Howard E Perry & Co. Ltd, England, a subsidiary of Klöckner & Co.KGaA, responsible for the area of finance, IT and administration.

1991 additionally General Manager of the subsidiary Hughes & Spencer Ltd, Stourbridge, England.

Multi-annual Chairman of the Economic and Tax Committee of the National Association of Steel Stockholders (NASS), Birmingham.

1992 self-employed as Managing Director and co-founder of the software company ProMet Systems Ltd.

2003 Returning to health care, such as volunteering within MIND, an organization providing care and counseling to people with mental illnesses such as schizophrenia, depression and other associated diseases.

Since 2004 in multi-annual series of several weeks of training and further education in authentic Ayurvedic healing, as well as introduction to Sanathana Sai Sanjeevini, a special kind of spiritual healing, by Sri C.R.Shastri, Chennai, Tamil Nadu, India.

Currently: Head of Ayurveda and naturopathic practice Lubeck, author of scientific publications, active as a speaker and seminar leader in the Federal Association "Free Naturopaths e.V." (Freie Heilpraktiker e.V., Berufs- und Fachverband)